Pocket Where There Is No Doctor: FIRST AID

Hesperian Health Guides

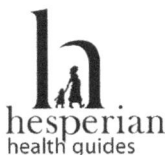

hesperian
health guides

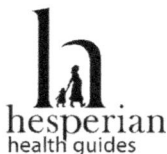

Published by:
Hesperian Health Guides
2860 Telegraph Avenue
Oakland, California 94609 USA
www.hesperian.org

THIS BOOK CAN BE IMPROVED WITH YOUR HELP.

If you are a community health worker, doctor, parent, or anyone with ideas or suggestions for ways this book could be changed to better meet the needs of your community, please write to Hesperian at the above address or email us at hesperian@ hesperian.org. Thank you for your help.

Contents

Establish Calm and Take Action

When an emergency happens, having a step-by-step approach can help you think clearly and care for the most important problems first.

1. Take a deep breath. Emergencies can be scary. But the calmer you are, the more helpful you can be. Being calm will also comfort and help the injured person or people around you.

2. Ask yourself: is this place safe? Move the person and yourself away from fires, busy streets, or other dangers. (If a person might have a neck or back injury, move them carefully so you do not move their neck. See pages 31 to 33.)

3. Try to be as gentle and comforting as you can, and explain what you're doing as you do it. If an injured person is awake and aware, ask their permission to touch them before you start to help. Injured people are often scared and in pain. When a person calms down, this helps to slow their fast heart beat and fast breathing.

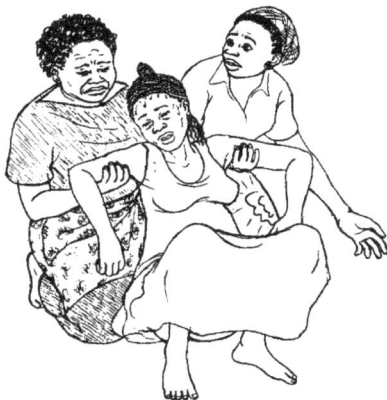

4. No matter what caused someone's injury, **check their breathing immediately.** It is the most important function needed for life. If the person is not breathing, check if their airway is blocked (page 8) and if the person needs rescue breathing (pages 10 to 11).

5. After breathing, **check for bleeding.** Heavy bleeding can kill. See page 14.

6. When the person is breathing and bleeding is controlled, check their whole body for other injuries and broken bones. Start at their head and check every part of the body, front and back, down to the toes. Gently ask questions, look the person over, and carefully touch their body to check for injuries you do not see at first. In an emergency, it is common for people to have more than one injury.

Protect yourself

Try to keep blood and other body fluids off yourself when caring for people who are injured. Do not touch anything soiled by body fluids with bare hands.

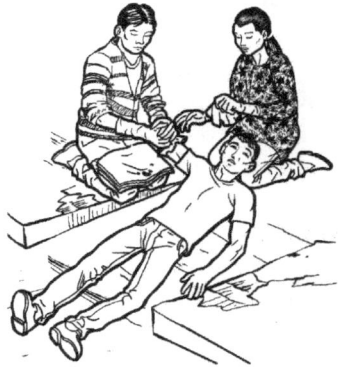

- **Cover your skin and eyes.** Wear clean gloves (plastic bags worn on your hands will work) and protective glasses if you can.
- **Wash your hands often, even if you wear gloves**. If body fluids get in your eyes or into open cuts on your skin, flush these to prevent infection.

Check the person's breathing often and make sure their bleeding is under control. Also check their blood pressure if you can. Regularly recheck these signs and keep talking to the person. This will help you notice if they become confused, or if their condition gets worse. See page 4 for what to do if this happens.

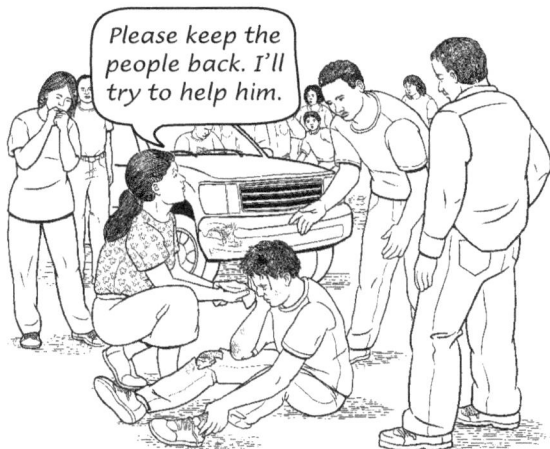

If people gather nearby, encourage them to help. Giving out tasks will keep people calm and help you support the injured person. Ask loud, assertive people to clear a space around you and the injured person. Have someone go for medical help and someone else get supplies like cloth (for bandages) or blankets.

The injured person can also help themself by putting pressure on their own wounds to stop bleeding (page 14). This can focus the person and allows you to check for other injuries or to care for other injured people.

When someone needs help:

? **Ask** if the person has pain, numbness, or difficulty moving.

➡ These are signs of sprains, broken ribs (page 36), or broken bones (page 40). If there is numbness or difficulty moving the lower body or the whole body, there may be a spinal cord injury (page 31).

➡ Stabbing pain when breathing may be a broken rib (page 36).

Ask or notice if they are having trouble breathing.

➡ A person who cannot cough or talk may be choking (page 8).

➡ Shortness of breath and wheezing can be signs of asthma (page 113). Trouble breathing can also be caused by chemical poisoning or drug overdose (pages 64 to 69).

Notice if they seem confused or have trouble speaking clearly. This can help you to assess how badly injured they are. See what to do If the person is unconscious (page 6).

➡ Many people become confused after an accident. But unclear speech, losing consciousness, and lasting confusion can be signs of head injury (pages 33 to 36) or intoxication from drugs or alcohol (pages 68 and 69).

➡ Slurred speech can be a sign of stroke. Check if one side of their face or body is drooping or weak. If they have these signs, get them to a hospital as soon as possible.

➡ Confusion or changes in consciousness can be a sign of a diabetic emergency (page 70).

? **Look** carefully for bleeding, swelling, bruises, redness, or disfigured body parts. Compare one side of the body to the other. For example, if one leg looks shorter, it may be broken.

➡ See what to do for bleeding (pages 14 to 16).

➡ Bruises, swelling, and disfigured body parts can be signs of broken bones (page 40).

➡ Bruising, swelling, and redness can also be signs of bleeding inside the body. Watch for shock (page 17).

? **Feel** gently along the head, face, neck, back, front, arms, and legs. Does the person have pain or numbness? Do you feel any bones out of place?

➡ Confusion, loss of consciousness, memory loss, nausea and vomiting, and blurred vision are signs of head injury (pages 33 to 36).

➡ Pain in the neck or back, weakness or loss of movement in the arms or legs, and numbness in the arms or legs are signs of a spinal cord injury (pages 31 to 33). Do not move the person.

Loss of Consciousness

Common causes of loss of consciousness are:

- shock (page 17)
- head injury (page 33)
- heart attack (page 39)
- stroke
- poisoning (page 64)
- blood sugar too low (page 70)
- seizures (page 73)
- heat stroke (page 82)
- too much alcohol, drugs, or medicine (page 68)

If a person is unconscious and you do not know why, immediately check each of the following:

1. Is he breathing well? If not, tilt his head way back and pull the jaw and tongue forward. If something is stuck in his throat, pull it out. If he is not breathing, use rescue breathing at once (pages 10 to 11).

2. If he might have a neck or back injury, do not move him because any change of position may cause greater injury. If you have to move him, do so with great care without bending his back or neck (page 31).

3. Is he losing a lot of blood? If so, try to stop the bleeding (page 14).

4. Is he in shock (moist, pale skin; weak, rapid pulse)? If so, lay him with his head lower than his feet and loosen his clothing (page 18).

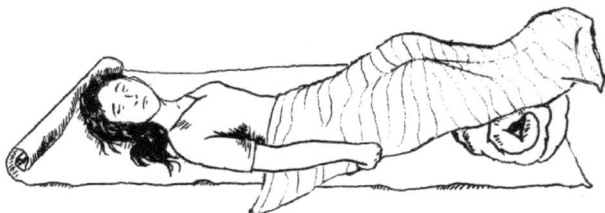

5. Could it be heat stroke (no sweat, high fever, hot, red skin)? If so, shade him from the sun, keep his head higher than his feet, soak him with cold water (ice water if possible), and fan him (page 81).

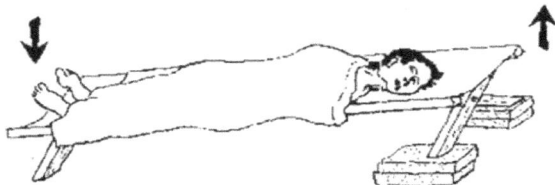

6. If he is breathing and you are sure there are no back or neck injuries, the person can be rolled to the side to prevent choking if he vomits.

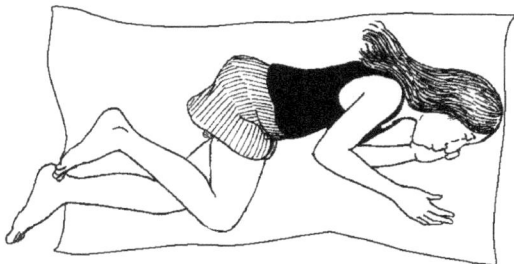

Never give anything by mouth to a person who is unconscious.

Breathing
Choking

When food or something else gets stuck in the throat or airway and a person cannot breathe, this is choking.

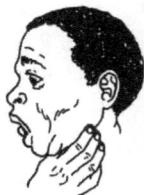

If the person is coughing, let them continue coughing but if they cannot talk or cannot cough, you can save a life by helping quickly.

Learn how to help a baby that is choking, see page 9.

Give back blows

Bend him over at the waist, and give 5 firm blows on the middle of the back, between the shoulder blades. Use the palm of your hand.

If this does not work:

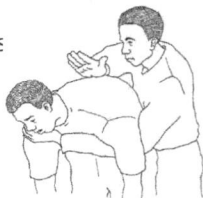

Give abdominal thrusts

Stand behind the person and wrap your arms around his waist

Put your fist against his belly, just above the navel and below the ribs.

Cover your fist with your other hand and use both hands to pull up and in with a sudden, strong jerk. Use enough force to lift the person off his feet. (Use less force on a small child.)

Repeat this 5 times in a row.

If there is something blocking air from getting to the lung or throat, the force of air being pushed so hard should drive it out.

For a pregnant woman or someone who is very fat, put your arms around the middle chest (put your fist between the breasts). Then thrust straight in.

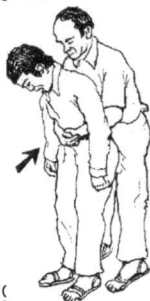

If the person is choking and becomes unconscious

Carefully lay him on his back and look in the mouth. If you can see food or something else blocking the throat, sweep it out with a hooked finger. But do not dig into the throat as this may drive the object in further. Then give rescue breathing (pages 10 to 11).

For a baby younger than one year

If a baby is choking and cannot cry or cough, try to clear her throat with back blows and chest thrusts.

Position the baby

Hold the baby face down with her head lower than her body.

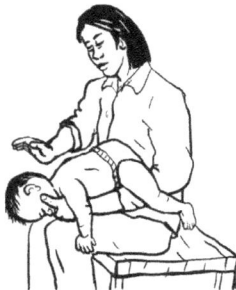

Give back blows

Use the heel of your hand to give 5 firm blows between the shoulder blades.

If the baby does not start breathing, turn her over.

Give chest thrusts

Put 2 or 3 fingers in the center of the chest – just below the nipples.

Use a firm, quick movement to push the chest down about 2 centimeters. Do this 5 times or until the baby breathes.

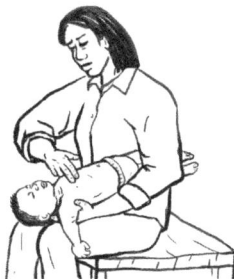

If you cannot clear the airway for a baby, child, or adult, give rescue breathing (pages 10 to 11).

Drowning

Get the person out of the water as fast as you can and immediately start rescue breathing (pages 10 to 11) and chest compressions (page 13). Give the rescue breaths first to get some air into the person's body.

If the person vomits, turn him on his side and gently use your finger or a cloth to wipe the vomit away so he does not choke on it.

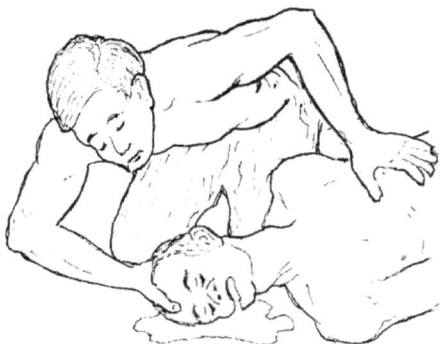

Rescue breathing

People can only live about 4 minutes without breathing. You may be able to save someone's life with rescue breaths if he stopped breathing because he choked, was hit on the head, almost drowned, was electrocuted, overdosed on drugs, or has hypothermia (extreme cold).

If a person stops breathing, you can save his life by giving rescue breathing immediately.

Postion his head

Lay the person face up. Lift the chin
and push on the forehead to tilt the
head back so his nose is pointing
straight up.

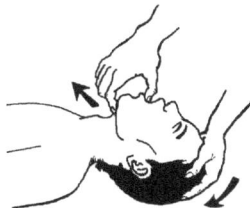

Give rescue breaths

Pinch his nose closed so air does
not escape that way.

Cover his mouth completely with yours.

Give 2 strong, slow breaths.

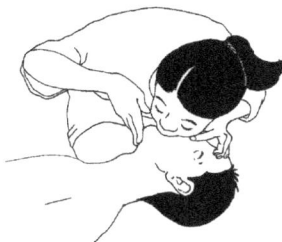

The chest should rise with each breath. If it does not,
the air is not getting into the lungs. Reposition the
head slightly and try again. Let the person breathe
out after each breath.

Check for a pulse

After 2 breaths, check if he is breathing.
Feel for a pulse on either side of the neck,
or listen to the chest, right over the heart.

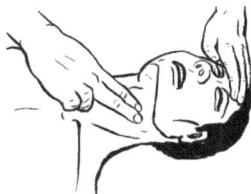

If there is no pulse, see "No Heartbeat" on the
next page.

If you do feel or hear a pulse, keep giving breaths
until he breathes on his own. It may take 30 minutes
or more.

No Heartbeat

Check for a pulse (sign of a heartbeat) on the neck (page 11). Or listen by putting your ear on the left side of the chest (where the drawing shows an X).

If there is no heartbeat, try to restart it with chest compressions. It is important to start chest compressions quickly, so if you are not sure if you have found a heartbeat, or if the heartbeat is very faint, it is safest to do chest compressions. (See instructions on page 13.)

This may bring life back to someone after electrocution, drowning, if he suffered a very hard blow to the chest, hypothermia (too cold), or drug overdose. Chest compressions are less likely to help someone after a heart attack, but are worth trying, especially if you cannot get more medical help. (See more about heart attacks on page 39.)

A medical device called a defibrillator gives an electric shock to re-start the heart after a heart attack. Find out before emergencies happen if there are defibrillators in your community and where they are kept. They are sometimes found in ambulances, or in public places like a police station or a large hotel.

Give chest compressions

Push hard and fast on the center of the chest 30 times.

Push straight down, about 5 cm (2 in).

Try for a fast rate, at least 100 times a minute, but the exact rate is not important.

Push hard and fast!

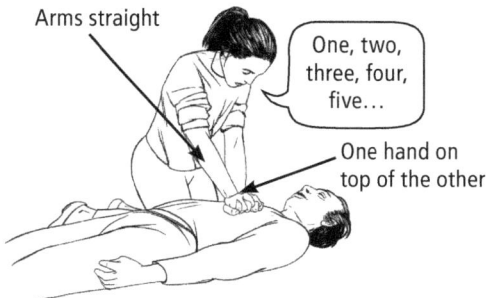

Arms straight

One, two, three, four, five…

One hand on top of the other

Give rescue breaths

After 30 chest compressions,

give 2 rescue breaths that make the chest rise (page 11).

Continue with compressions and breaths

Keep alternating between 30 chest compressions and 2 rescue breaths. You may have to do this for a long time. Continue until the person is breathing and alert, or until there is no doubt he is dead.

Get help

If you can get the person to a hospital quickly, do so.

Keep giving chest compressions and rescue breathing on the way.

This will help to keep the body functions going until you can get help.

Bleeding

Direct pressure

Direct, firm pressure will stop almost all bleeding, even large, heavily bleeding wounds. If the person is bleeding from the head, apply pressure and see page 35.

1. Raise the injured part so it is above the level of the person's heart.

2. Grab the cleanest piece of cloth you can find nearby, fold it to about the size of the wound, and press it directly and firmly on the wound. Show the injured person how to put pressure on himself, if he is able. If the wound is large, put the gauze or cloth into the wound. Keep pressing until the bleeding stops. Do not remove the cloth if it becomes soaked with blood. Instead, add another cloth on top. For a large wound, do not lift your hand off until at least 15 minutes has passed, even to check if it has stopped bleeding.

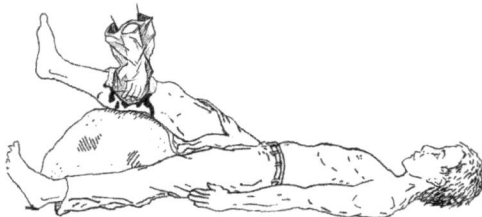

When bleeding has slowed or stopped, you may be able to wrap a dressing firmly around the bleeding part. Put a folded piece of gauze or cloth in or on top of the wound and then firmly wrap a bandage around it. Be sure the bandage is firm enough to create pressure on the wound, but not so tight that it cuts off the blood flow to the rest of the arm or leg.

Applying pressure to stop bleeding is hard work.. Do not give up!

Never use dirt, kerosene, lime, or used coffee grounds to stop bleeding.

Blood can make a big mess and look like the person lost more than he did. But watch the person closely for these signs of losing too much blood:

DANGER SIGNS
- Confusion or losing consciousness
- Very fast heart rate
- Cold, moist, pale skin

If you see these signs, raise both the person's feet onto something so they are above the heart, and get help for shock (page 17).

Even if you do not see these signs, stay with the person or check in on him every 10 to 15 minutes to make sure he is OK and reassure him. Keep checking until he is acting and feeling normal.

Tourniquets

Use a tourniquet **only as a last resort,** when you are willing to risk the loss of an arm or leg in order to save a person's life.

Use tourniquets only when:
- **A limb is cut off** or is so mangled that it clearly cannot be saved.
- **There is heavy bleeding that does not slow down from an arm or leg** with direct pressure. (Have you tried pressing harder first?)
- **There is a large, deep wound in the thigh,** like when a bullet, shrapnel, or something else has penetrated deep into the muscle, and the person is showing signs of blood loss like weakness, confusion, or pale skin. (It can be impossible to use enough pressure on a large thigh to stop heavy bleeding.)

Use a wide belt, a piece of cloth folded into a flat strip, or a blood pressure cuff inflated all the way to tie off the bleeding part. Do not use thin string or wire. It will cut right through the skin.

Get to a hospital as fast as you can. You have 2 or 3 hours before the limb is likely to be lost.

Step 1:

Place the tourniquet **above but close** to the wound, between the wound and the body. (A common mistake is putting the tourniquet too far from the wound.)

Step 2:

Wrap the tourniquet tightly around the limb twice. Then tie a knot.

Step 3:

Put a short, strong stick on top of the knot. Tie two more knots on top of the stick.

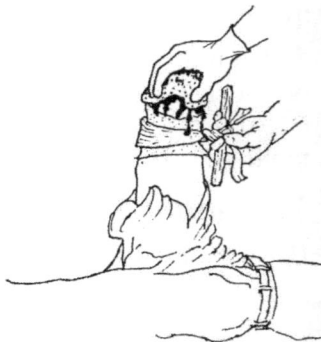

Step 4:

Twist the stick to tighten the tourniquet until bleeding stops.

Step 5:

Tie the stick in place with another cloth.

Shock

Shock is a life-threatening condition that can result from severe bleeding, dehydration, major wounds and burns, allergic reaction, or infection in the blood (sepsis). This kind of shock is different from "shock" from a surprise or scare. The body starts to shut down, losing the ability to perform its most basic functions. Once signs of shock begin, it tends to get worse very fast. Treat shock quickly to save the person's life.

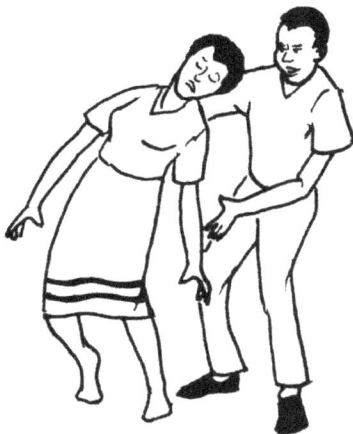

SIGNS

- Fear or restlessness, then confusion, weakness, and loss of consciousness
- Cold sweat
- Weak, fast
- Dropping l

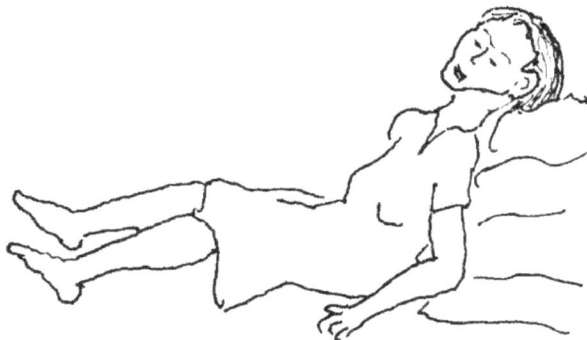

TREATMENT

Get help. On the way:

- Treat the cause of the shock as quickly as you can:
  - » For bleeding, use pressure (page 14).
  - » For dehydration, the person will need fluids by IV if she cannot sit up and swallow liquids.
  - » If the cause of shock is sepsis (an infection that has spread to the bloodstream), antibiotics are needed immediately (page 28).
- Keep the person warm (or remove some clothes if the person is hot).
- Raise the legs, supporting the knees.
- Keep calm and reassure the person.

Wounds

1. Stop the bleeding with pressure (page 14).
2. Clean the wound thoroughly as soon as you can. The better you clean it, the less likely it is to become infected. For larger wounds, give some kind of pain medicine before you clean and care for the wound. Inject lidocaine (page 124) around the wound and just below the skin inside it. Or give another pain medicine and allow time for it to work.
3. Dress or close the wound, or for a small wound, leave it open to heal.

Clean all wounds

*Any wound, big or small, can become infected.
Clean every wound well.*

Wash your hands well with soap. Then wash the wound with 1 to 4 liters of flowing water. You do not need antiseptics, some of which can slow healing down. If the wound looks dirty, use soapy water and then rinse that off with plain water.

Lift up any flaps of skin to clean underneath. For deep wounds, squirt the inside of the wound with a bulb syringe, letting the water run out.

Or take the needle off a syringe and squirt water into the wound.

Or just run lots of clean water over and into the wound.

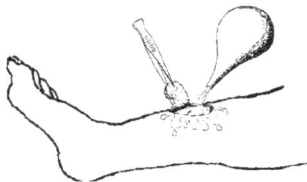

Wash out anything left inside the wound, especially dirt, wood, or other rough material. You may need to use a piece of sterile gauze or clean fabric to clean out the wound, then rinse thoroughly.

Caring for wounds

As the wound heals, make sure it stays clean to prevent
infection. If it gets dirty, clean the wound with lots of water.
Covering the wound with a bandage, sterile gauze, washed
banana leaf, or very clean piece of cloth will help keep it clean.
Putting honey on the wound also helps prevent infection.
Change the bandage daily, and if it becomes wet or dirty. It is
better to have no bandage than one that is dirty or wet.

Watch for signs of infection such as increasing redness,
pain, heat, swelling, bad smell, or pus at the site of the wound.
For any of these signs, clean the wound well. You may need
to gently pull open the wound to clean it. Watch that the
infection does not spread to other parts of the body (page 27).

Closing wounds

A small wound is best left alone to heal. It should not need
stitches. The most important thing is to keep wounds clean.

A wound that is more than 12 hours old should be cleaned
and left open to heal.

A larger wound that comes together well will heal better if
it is closed.

To close a shallow, clean wound, use butterfly bandages,
glue, or stitches.

Butterfly bandage

Use a butterfly bandage for a small cut.

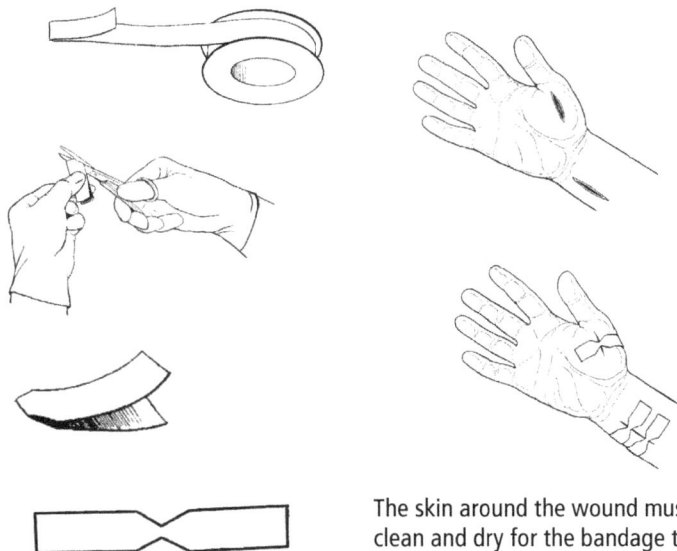

The skin around the wound must be clean and dry for the bandage to stick.

Glue

Super Glue or *Krazy Glue* (cyanoacrylate, a powerful adhesive) is easier to use than sutures and works just as well for most wounds. Use it when you can clearly see how the two sides of the wound should go together. It may not work as well on hands or joints because they move so much. Do not use glue near the eyes or mouth. *Super Glue* may irritate the skin.

Step 1:

Make sure the wound is clean
and the skin around it is dry.

Step 2:

Push the sides of the wound together.
Keep fingers well away from the wound
so they do not stick to the glue.
A helper can use a couple of clean
sticks to hold the sides together.

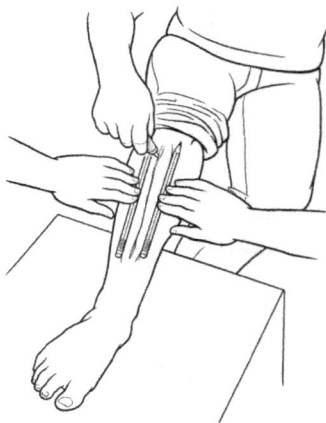

Step 3:

Squeeze a line of glue along
the closed edges of the wound.

Step 4:

Hold the wound closed for 30 seconds. Then add another layer of glue. Wait another 30 seconds or so, and then add a third layer. Each layer should cover a little more of the surrounding skin than the last.

The glue will wear away on its own. By then the wound should be healed.

Stitches (sutures)

A cut will benefit from stitches if it is shallow and long, or if the edges of the skin around the cut do not come together by themselves.

Line up the edges. The edges of the wound should come up slightly above the skin instead of tucking into the wound.

Make the depth and the length of the stitch the same on each side of the wound.

Step 1:

Put the stitch through the cut, not under the cut.

Put the stitch through here

not here

If you do not have suture or a curved suturing needle, sharpen a sewing needle. Sterilize the needle, some silk or nylon thread, and a small pair of pliers for pulling the needle through tough skin. To sterilize these tools, bake them at 170°C (340°F) for 1 hour or 150°C (305°F) for 2½ hours. If you cannot sterilize the tools you have, close the wound with glue instead (page 22).

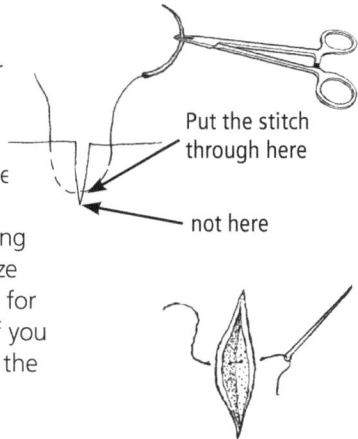

Step 2:

Tie a secure knot. See "How to tie a strong knot" on the next page.

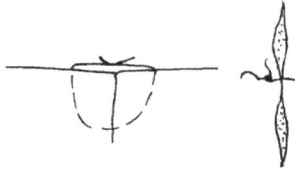

Step 3:

Make enough stitches to close the whole cut.

A deep wound should get a couple of stitches inside the muscle with dissolvable sutures before sewing the skin together. If you cannot do this then do not close the wound.

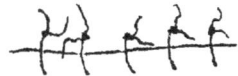

How to tie a strong knot:

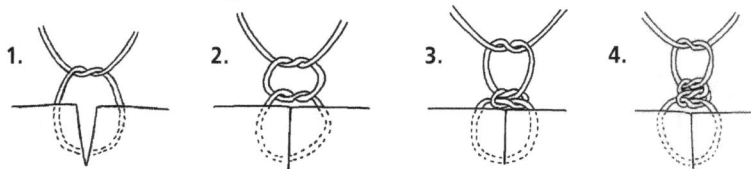

1.   2.   3.   4.

Leave stitches in place for about one week (10 days for a leg or joint wound). Then cut each stitch and pull it out. If you spend some time sewing clothes, you will find that your skill to suture wounds improves as well.

Deep Wounds

Deep wounds should generally be left open to heal. Wounds that are not closed properly can easily become infected. Rough, messy wounds and puncture wounds in particular should be cleaned twice a day with boiled water and kept open, or re-opened, so they will heal from the inside.

Deep wounds can develop a tetanus infection, see page 29. Unless the person had a tetanus vaccination within the last 5 years, they will need one now and also an injection of antitetanus immunoglobulin (pages 104 to 107).

If you are not sure whether closing a wound is a good idea, it probably is not.

*Never close animal bites, puncture wounds,
or rough, messy wounds.*

Animal bites

Clean animal bites very well with soap
and water for 15 minutes or more.
Animal bites are likely to get infected,
so give amoxicillin with clavulanic acid
(page 91) or another combination of
antibiotics for animal bites. For monkey, bat, and raccoon bites,
get a rabies vaccination and immunoglobulin immediately. Do
the same for dog bites if the dog could have rabies. See page 108
for more about medicines for animal bites.

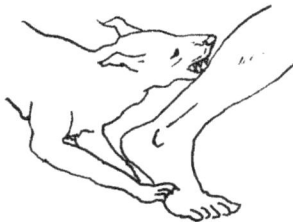

Rabies is deadly. It affects the brain causing signs like
confusion or paralysis. Then, in just a few days, the person
becomes unconscious leading to death. Following a bite from
an animal with rabies, it can take a month or a few months for
signs to appear but by then it is too late to treat. If you think
rabies is a possibility and do not have rabies vaccine or rabies
immunoglobulin, contact your local health authority as soon as
possible after the bite.

Even if there is no rabies immunoglobulin available, washing
the skin thoroughly right away with soap and repeated rinsing,
and giving the series of rabies vaccine as soon as possible can
prevent rabies.

Knife wounds

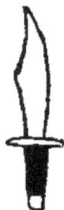

Deep knife wounds should usually be kept open and
cleaned often. Give cloxacillin (page 92), clindamycin
(page 98), or cephalexin (page 102) at any sign of
infection.

Knife wounds to the chest or belly can be very
dangerous. Get medical help. Know what to do on the
way for a knife wound to the chest (page 36), or a knife
wound to the belly (page 37).

Gunshot Wounds

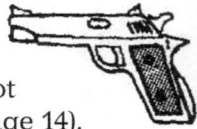

Get medical help as soon as possible for gunshot wounds. Stop bleeding with direct pressure (page 14). Check both where the bullet entered and where it exited. If there is no exit wound, the bullet may have to be removed.

Gunshot wounds are likely to become infected. In all cases, wash the wound well and give one of these: cloxacillin, clindamycin, or cephalexin.

For a bullet in the head, on the way to get help, raise the head a little with folded blankets or pillows. Cover the wound with a clean bandage.

If there is any chance that the bullet hit a bone, the bone may be cracked or broken through. Splint the limb and do not use it for several weeks. See pages 40 to 46.

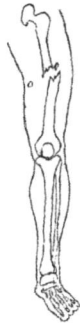

Fish hooks

Step 1:

Push the hook through the skin so it pokes out the other side like this:

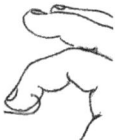

Step 2:

Cut off the barb or the shank.

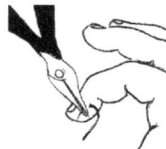

Step 3:

Pull the rest of the hook out.

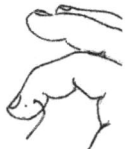

Infection

Any wound can become infected.

SIGNS OF INFECTION

The wound is infected if it:
- becomes swollen, red, hot, and painful
- has pus
- begins to smell bad

The infection is spreading to other parts of the body if:
- it causes fever
- the lymph nodes become swollen and tender

Lymph nodes are little traps for germs that form small lumps under the skin when a nearby part of the body has an infection. Swollen lymph nodes mean infection.

Behind the ear means an infection on the head or scalp, often caused by sores or lice. Or German measles (rubella) may be the cause.

Below the jaw means infection of the teeth or throat.

Below the ear and on the neck means infection of the ear, face, or head. Or it could be tuberculosis.

In the armpit means an infection of the arm, head, or breast. Or sometimes breast cancer.

In the groin means an infection of the leg, foot, genitals,

TREATMENT FOR INFECTION

Clean the wound well. You may need to open up an abscess
or remove stitches. Unless the infected area is small, shows
no signs of infection, and is healing quickly, it is usually wise
to give antibiotics. Give dicloxacillin (page 93), cephalexin
(page 102), or clindamycin (page 98). A person who is not
up-to-date with tetanus vaccinations needs a vaccination
and, if the wound is deep, also an injection of antitetanus
immunoglobulin (pages 104 to 107).

If the infection does not get better, it can spread through
the blood. This is called sepsis.

Sepsis

Sepsis is when an infection spreads to the bloodstream. It is
dangerous because it can lead to shock. If you suspect sepsis,
get medical help quickly and treat the person on the way.

SIGNS OF SEPSIS

- Fever or too low temperature
- Fast heart rate—pulse is more than 90 beats per
  minute
- Fast breathing—more than 20 breaths
  per minute
- Difficulty breathing
- Splotchy or pale skin
- Less urine
- Confusion or losing consciousness
- Low blood pressure

The most important signs are fever or
too low temperature, fast heart rate, and fast breathing. If the
person has 2 or more of these signs, treat for sepsis.

TREATMENT

Get medical help. On the way:

- Watch for and treat any signs of shock (page 17).
- Give ceftriaxone (page 101), OR ciprofloxacin (page 100) plus clindamycin (page 98).
- Clean any infected wounds, remove dead skin, and if you know how, drain abscesses of pus.
- If the person is breathing well, give fluids to drink. Give small sips frequently.

Tetanus (lockjaw)

Tetanus is a deadly infection that gets into a wound and then spreads throughout the body.

SIGNS

Signs of tetanus most often appear 7 to 10 days after an injury. But signs can also start as soon as 3 days after being infected or not appear until 2 or 3 weeks later.

- Tense and painful contractions of all the muscles.
- During contractions, breathing may stop.
- Extreme muscle spasms that come and go.
- Lockjaw (cannot open the mouth easily).
- Stiff neck and a stiff, board-hard belly.

Get medical help fast for these signs!

Tetanus is much easier to prevent than to treat. Prevent by vaccinating all children against tetanus and carefully cleaning wounds so they do not get infected. Children need 3 doses of the tetanus vaccine as infants and then 3 booster vaccines later (page 106). Pregnant women need a tetanus vaccination unless they have had one recently.

Wounds most likely to develop tetanus

- Animal bites, especially those of dogs and pigs.
- Puncture wounds (from thorns, splinters, nails, or other sharp objects).
- Gunshot wounds.
- Broken bones, when the bone pokes through the skin (open fractures).
- Severe burns or frostbite.
- Any procedure that cuts into the skin, using tools that have not been sterilized.

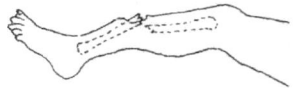

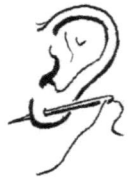

Deep or dirty wounds need special cleaning, care, and antibiotics (pages 24 to 26). Unless the person had a tetanus vaccine within the past 5 years, they need one now and also an injection of antitetanus immunoglobulin (pages 104 to 107).

Newborn tetanus

Newborns can get infected with tetanus when unsterilized tools are used to cut the umbilical cord at birth, or when the cord stump is not kept clean and dry afterward. Cutting the cord with a sterilized blade, keeping the stump clean, and making sure the mother has an up-to-date tetanus vaccination (page 106) protects the baby from tetanus at and right after birth.

If a newborn has signs of tetanus, get them medical help right away. If the hospital or health center is more than 2 hours away and you know how, give benzathine benzylpenicillin (page 94) on the way.

Back and Neck Injuries

Inside the bones of the back is the spinal cord, an extension of the brain. An injury to the spinal cord can cause life-long disability or death. If there is any chance the person injured their spinal cord, you can protect them from further injury by **keeping their neck and back still!**

Assume that the spinal cord may be injured after any car, motorcycle, or bicycle crash, any big fall, or blow to the back or head. Keep the neck and back still so they cannot turn side to side or up and down. Tape a roll of clothes, fabric, foam, or something similar around the neck to keep it from moving.

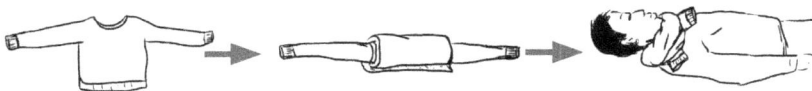

Do not give pain medicine until you are sure there is no injury to the spinal cord. Pain reminds the person to keep still.

SIGNS OF SPINAL CORD INJURY

- Pain or tenderness along the neck or back
- Weakness or loss of movement in the arms or legs
- Numbness in the arms or legs

Other signs of spinal cord injury include loss of control of urine or stool, difficulty breathing, or shock (page 17). If there is any doubt, it is safest to treat the person as if they have a spinal cord injury.

To check for spinal cord injury, ask the person to stay flat on their back and to raise their knees. Then ask them to raise their arms. Can they move without difficulty? Do they feel pain? Touch their fingers and toes. Can they feel your touch? Can they feel your pinch?

If there is a place on the body below which the person cannot move or feel, they likely have a spinal cord injury. With help from others, you can prevent this injury from getting worse.

If the person has feeling and movement in all of their body, carefully "log roll" them to their side to check their whole back.

Keep the head, neck, and back in one straight line as you roll. Then keep the body still, and gently feel each bump along the person's back, in a line, from the back of the head to just above the buttocks. Feel for bones that are broken or out of place, and notice if the person shows signs of feeling pain (for example, crying out).

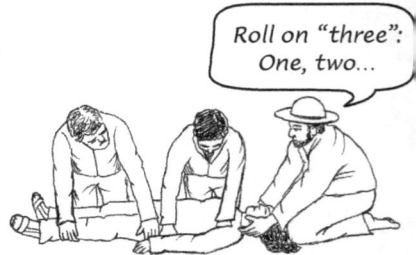

Roll on "three": One, two...

Hold the head in line with the body, keep the neck straight.

Use the same group effort to carefully roll the person back.

(If the person is vomiting, place something under their head so they can stay on their side.)

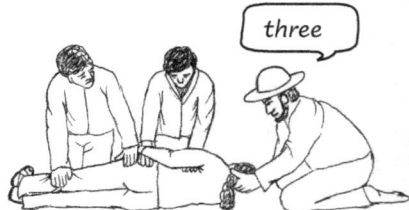

three

If there is pain or tenderness, the person needs x-rays to see if there are smaller breaks in the bones. They will need to rest in one position, being turned every few hours but keeping the neck and back still, until pain subsides in a week or so.

To move the person, log roll them onto their side and put a long flat board, like a wooden door, under them. Then roll them back onto the board. Use a few long strips of strong tape or cloth to secure their head, chest, and thighs to the board. If you must keep the person on this board for a long time, you should roll them to their side every couple of hours.

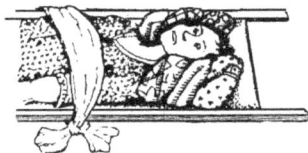

A person who has had an injury to the spine needs long-term physical therapy. Seek help from those with experience, or use a book like *Disabled Village Children* or *A Health Handbook for Women with Disabilities,* both available from Hesperian.

Head Injuries

If someone falls, gets hit in the head, or is in a vehicle accident, watch for signs of brain injury. It can be difficult to tell if there is brain injury if the person has been drinking or using drugs because many of these signs can be the same. Also check anyone with a head injury for neck or back injuries (page 31), as these two can go together.

SIGNS OF A MILD BRAIN INJURY OR CONCUSSION

- Confusion or loss of consciousness that gets better on its own in a short time
- Not remembering what happened
- Temporary blurry vision or "seeing stars"
- Nausea or vomiting that does not last long
- Headache, dizziness, or tiredness

Ask the person to rest for about 24 hours and give paracetamol (acetaminophen) for the pain, but do not give ibuprofen or aspirin because they can worsen any bleeding inside the head. Watch the person for the first 24 hours. If she goes to sleep, wake her every few hours to see if she can still answer questions and think clearly. In the hours after the injury, if the person becomes more confused, gets a headache that gets worse and worse, or loses consciousness or has a seizure, there is likely bleeding inside the skull and immediate medical help is needed.

SIGNS OF SEVERE BRAIN INJURY

Get help for any of these signs:

- Unconsciousness
- Severe or worsening headache, changes in vision, loss of balance
- Nausea and vomiting
- Confusion, personality changes, aggression
- Very slow, very fast, or changing (irregular) heartbeat
- Fast, shallow breathing or breathing that is irregular (sometimes fast, sometimes slow)
- Warm, flushed skin
- Seizures
- Blood or clear fluid leaking from the ears or nose

These signs may happen hours after the injury:
• One pupil bigger than the other
• Bruises around both eyes or behind the ear

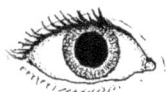

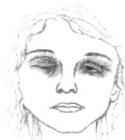

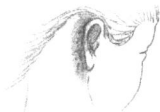

Bleeding from the head

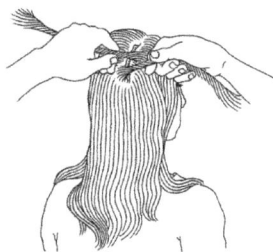

Head wounds bleed a lot. If you are sure the spine is not injured, ask the person to sit up, or prop her up, to decrease bleeding. Use pressure to stop the bleeding, then wash the wound well before closing it with sutures or glue. If you have no supplies you can tie the hair together across the wound, to help keep it closed, like this:

If the head is cut open, look for injury to the skull underneath. If you believe there may be an opening into the skull, apply pressure on each side of the wound and avoid pressing hard on the injured part of the head.

Nosebleeds

Pinch the nose firmly, just below the hard bony part.

Hold tight for 10 minutes—do not stop to check if the bleeding has stopped or the blood can start flowing again. If the nose still bleeds after 10 minutes, try pinching for another 10 minutes.

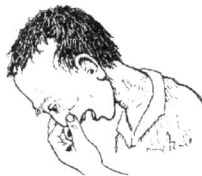

While most nosebleeds get better, any uncontrolled bleeding is dangerous. Beware especially of nose bleeds in old people.

36

PREVENTION
Rubbing a little petroleum jelly inside the nose might keep
dryness from causing bleeding. Nose picking is a common
cause of nosebleeds.

Chest Wounds and Broken Ribs

Tenderness to the touch, or
stabbing pain with breathing or
coughing after an injury to the
chest may be a broken rib. Feel
along the rib with your fingers.
If there is a spot where it sticks

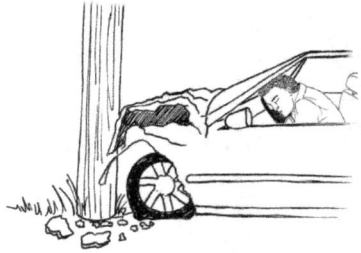

A fall or crushing injury can
break many ribs at once.

up under the skin, or where it dips in and is very tender, it
is broken. If only one rib is broken and it is not poking in or
out of the body, give pain medicine. The person should avoid
lifting and hard work for a few weeks. It will heal without any
special treatment. Remind person to take deep breaths every
few hours. This hurts, but keeps the lungs working.

Many broken ribs (flail chest)

1. Tape a thick pad, or folded piece of clothing over the
   broken ribs.

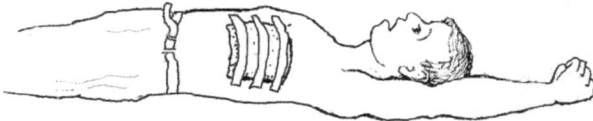

2. Lay the person in whatever position best helps breathe.
3. Watch for signs of shock (page 17) and get help.

Deep chest wounds

A gunshot, stab wound, explosion, or badly broken rib can cause air to leak in and out of the lungs.

1. Immediately cover the opening with anything airtight, like a bandage covered in petroleum jelly, a folded plastic bag, or a banana leaf.

2. Tape only 3 sides so air can get out but not get in.

3. Lay the person in whatever position best helps them breathe. Get help.

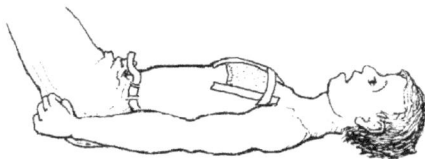

Abdomen Injuries and Wounds

If the belly has suffered a blow, such as from a hard fall, vehicle accident, or getting hit or kicked, look for bruises which are signs of bleeding trapped in the body. Too much bleeding inside the body can lead to shock.

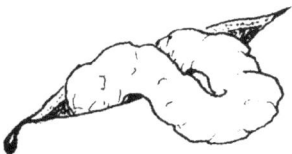

If part of the gut spills out of the body, cover it with a clean cloth soaked in lightly salted water and get help. Do not push the guts back in.

38

DANGER SIGNS
- Severe pain
- Confusion
- Belly hard like a board, or growing larger
- Signs of blood loss: feeling faint, growing pale, fast pulse

These are signs of serious injury to the abdomen. For any of these danger signs, treat for shock (page 17) and get help. Do not give any food or drink.

An object sticking out of the body

For an object sticking out of the abdomen, it is usually safest to leave it in and get help. Even if help is days away, do not pull out the object. Secure it in place with bandages or fabric.

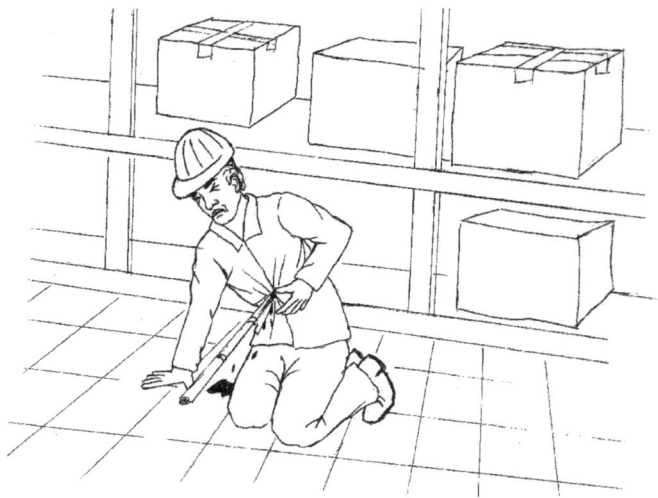

Heart Attack

Both men and women have heart attacks. Heart attack happens when blood flow to the heart is blocked for a long enough time that part of the heart muscle begins to die. This is usually caused by heart disease.

SIGNS

- Pressure, squeezing, tightness, burning, pain, or a full feeling in the chest
- The pain may spread to the neck, shoulder, arms, teeth, or jaw
- The pain usually comes on gradually, but sometimes can be sudden and intense
- Shortness of breath
- Sweating
- Nausea
- Feeling lightheaded

Chest pain is the most common sign for both men and women, **but women more often do not feel chest pain.** Instead they feel shortness of breath, tiredness, nausea, vomiting, or back or jaw pain.

TREATMENT

Give 1 tablet of aspirin right away (300 to 325 mg). Ask the person to chew it up and swallow it with water. Even if you are not sure the person is having a heart attack, aspirin will do no harm.

If you have it, give nitroglycerin dissolved under the tongue (page 114). Morphine helps with the pain and fear (page 123). Reassure the person and get help.

Broken Bones, Dislocations, and Sprains

First decide if the bone is broken or dislocated (out of joint), or if there is a sprain to ligaments that connect the bones. It can be very hard to tell these injuries apart, and an x-ray may be necessary to know for sure. If you cannot tell if it is broken, dislocated, or sprained, keep the body part still and get help. It is also possible to have a combination of these injuries.

Give paracetemol (acetaminophen) or ibuprofen to help with the pain.

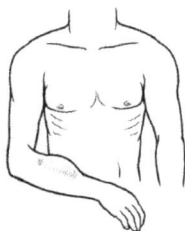

Broken

Mis-shapen in the middle of a bone or pain at one specific point on the bone, and little or no pain when it is kept still. Sometimes a bone could be broken even without being mis-shapen. An x-ray can tell you for sure if there is

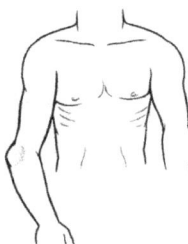

Dislocated

Deformed at a joint or unable to move a joint.

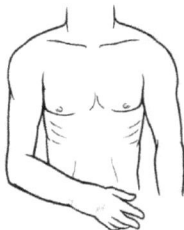

Sprain or Strain

Swelling and pain near a joint.

Broken bones

Keep a broken bone still until someone with experience setting bones can set it and put on a cast. To help keep it still, make a splint from a folded piece of cardboard, a flat piece of board, the stiff spine of a palm frond, or something else straight and hard.

Make a splint

Step 1:
Position the arm in its natural, resting position. The elbow should be bent.

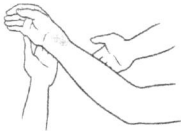

Step 2:
Wrap a layer of bandage, gauze, or thin cloth or use a shirt sleeve.

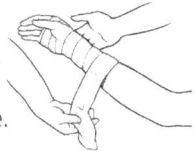

Step 3:
Pull the more distant part with a slow, steady, strong force. Do not yank, but pull hard enough to separate the bones.

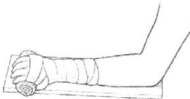

Step 4:
Wrap around the splint with a bandage or strip of fabric to hold it in place.

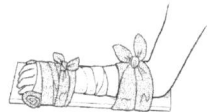

Leave fingers and toes uncovered and check often that they are warm and have normal feeling.

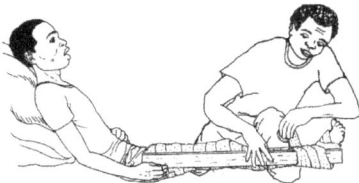

Splint a broken thigh bone from the hip all the way down to the ankle.

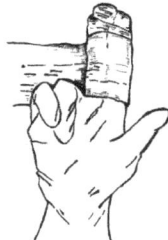

Splint a finger or toe to the one next to it. Put a little soft padding in between them.

Make a sling

You can use a sling to protect and support a wounded arm or
shoulder.

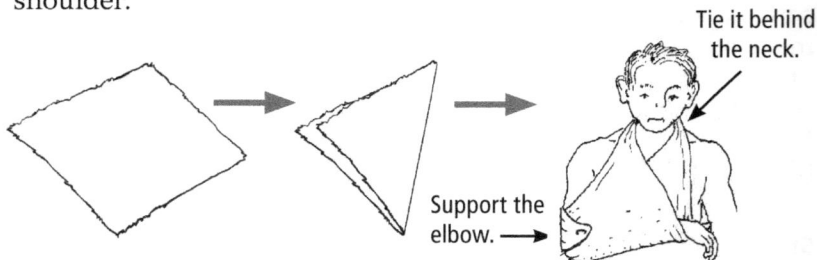

Tie it behind
the neck.

Support the
elbow. →

Set a bone

If the bone is out of its natural position, setting it will help
it heal. But if you do not know how to set a bone correctly,
you can cause a lot of damage by doing it wrong. Find an
experienced bonesetter or community health worker who
knows how to do this well.

Step 1:

First give pain medicine (page 119). You can also give an anti-anxiety
medicine like lorazepam or diazepam to help the person stay calm
(pages 124 to 126).

Step 2:

Ask a helper to hold the part close to the body still or tie it to
something that will not move.

Step 3:

Pull the more distant part with a slow,
steady, strong force. Do not yank, but
pull hard enough to separate the bones.

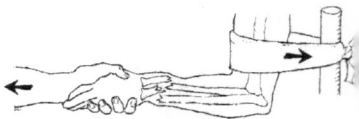

Step 4:

When the pieces of bone are separated, gently line up the two edges and let them come back together.

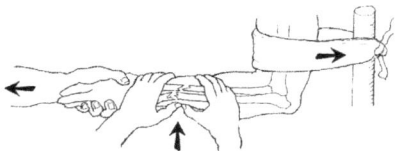

Do not try to set a bone if the break seems to go into the joint or if there seems to be more than one break, leaving a "floating" piece of bone in the middle. Do not jerk or force the bones in place.

Make a cast

Casts can be made from pieces of cloth and a syrup or plaster mix that dries hard.

In Mexico several different plants such as tepeguaje (a tree of the bean family) and solda con solda (a huge, tree-climbing arum lily) are used to make casts. In India, traditional bone-setters make casts using a mixture of egg whites and herbs. The methods are similar. Any plant will do if a syrup can be made from it that will dry hard and firm and will not irritate the skin. Usually the plant is boiled in water until a thick syrup forms. Or use plaster of Paris mixed with water.

Wait until the swelling has gone down before casting. This can take up to a week. In the meantime, support the limb with a splint and sling.

Step 1:

Make sure the bones are aligned. Compare the injured side to the uninjured side to make sure both look and feel the same.

Step 2:

Position an injured elbow so it is bent, with the thumb up, and fingers slightly curved—as if holding a glass.

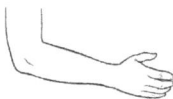

Position a knee so it is slightly bent. The ankle is bent as if the person were standing up.

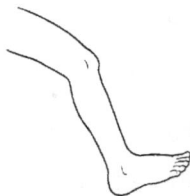

Step 3:

Wrap the area to be casted in a loose, thin layer of cloth or a few layers of gauze. Cast an area that includes the joint above and below the break.

Step 4:

Then wrap in soft cotton or kapok. Give extra padding to bony parts, but do not over-pad, especially around the broken part.

Step 5:

Dip strips of flannel, clean sheets, or bandages in the syrup or plaster mixture.

Step 6:

Form a cast around the area with layers of bandage. Leave fingers and toes uncovered. Keep the cast snug but not tight.

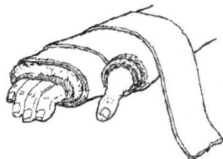

Step 7:

Smooth the inner wrapping over the edge of the cast, like this:

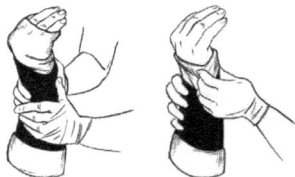

After the cast is on, rest the limb and keep it elevated when possible. Use crutches to avoid putting any weight on a broken leg.

If, at any time after the cast is on, the fingers or toes start to swell, feel more pain, turn red, pale, or blue, or lose feeling, **remove the cast immediately.** Failing to cut off a cast that is too tight can cause the person to lose the limb.

How long does a broken bone take to heal? A young child heals in a few weeks. An old person's bones take months and may never heal properly

Keep a cast on the arm for at least a month. Leg casts should stay on for about 2 months.

To remove the cast, soak it in water and carefully cut it off. After the cast is removed, be gentle with the broken limb for the same amount of time as the cast was on. Slowly start normal activities, such as putting weight on an injured leg.

Bone broken through the skin (open fractures)

Open fractures are very likely to become infected. Give one of the following: ceftriaxone, cloxacillin, clindamycin, or cephalexin, and get help.

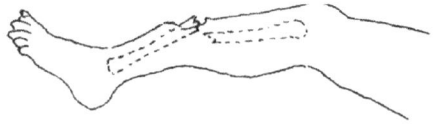

If you will be able to get to medical help within a few hours, wash your hands, and clean the wound very well with lots of flowing water for 5 minutes or more. Without putting the bone back under the skin, splint the limb.

If you know you cannot get to help within about 5 hours, clean the wound and bone ends without touching them. You may be able to help the bone go back to its position under the skin by pulling the limb in a straight line very gently (see "Set a bone,"page 42).

Do not use force and do not continue if the person says it is hurting more. Then dress the wound lightly in sterile gauze. Change the gauze often to avoid infection until the person can be treated by an experienced health worker. If you need to move the person, make a splint first to keep the limb in the same position (page 42).

Dislocations (bone out of the joint)

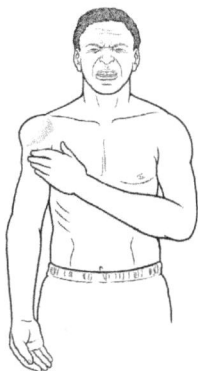

Re-set a dislocated bone as soon as you can. The longer you wait, the more difficult and painful it will be to fix. If you cannot get the bone back in the joint, splint to hold still in the position that feels most comfortable, and get help.

A person with experience may know how to pull the bone gently and slowly away from the joint, then let it "pop" back in correctly. Often when a bone comes out of the joint, pain and trauma make the muscles around it tighten which can prevent the bone from returning to the joint. Helping the person calm down and relax their muscles, and using an anti-anxiety medicine such as diazepam, and a pain medicine such as ibuprofen, can make resetting a dislocation possible.

After resetting a dislocated joint, keep it still for 2 or 3 weeks with a brace or sling. Use a general pain medicine such as ibuprofen as needed. As soon as the pain has lessened enough to allow movement, take the joint out of the sling every few hours and gently flex or rotate it. For a shoulder, hang the arm down and let it move back and forth and in small circles. Be gentle with the joint for the following 2 or 3 months. Dislocations take a long time to heal.

*If pain is severe after resetting a dislocated joint,
there may be a broken bone.*

Dislocated shoulder

Have the person lie
face down on a table
or surface that is
high enough that the
dislocated arm can
hang down without
touching the ground.
Ask the person to hold
a bucket with 5 to 7
liters (1 to 2 gallons)

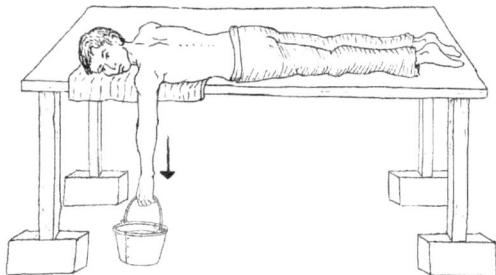

of water for 20 to 30 minutes. Tying an object weighing 3 to
5 kilos (5 to 10 pounds) to the person's wrist with a soft cloth
works too. This will tire the muscles so they relax, pull the
arm down, and allow the shoulder to go back into place.

If the shoulder does not go back into place, gently but
firmly push on the tip of the scapula (wing bones) with your
thumb. The arm should "clunk" back into place.

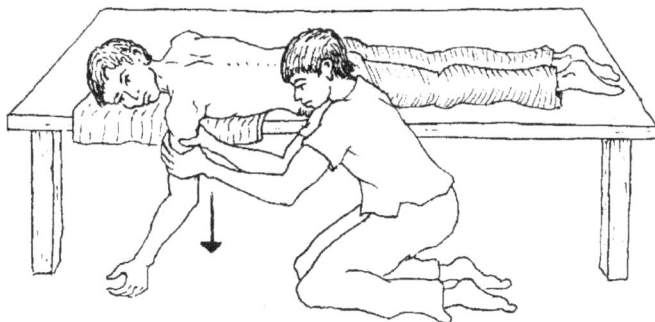

48

A different method is to have the person lie face up. Slowly rotate the arm toward you like this. It is best to have a helper holding the person's body still, so that just the arm moves.

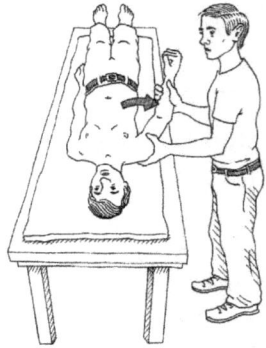

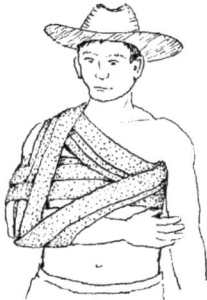

After, sling the arm like this to prevent it from slipping out of the joint again.

Dislocated elbow

Step 1:

Have the person lie down, then place the forearm straight in line with the upper arm to line up the bones.

Step 2:

Have a helper firmly hold the upper arm. Pull the forearm towards you, and gently bend the elbow.

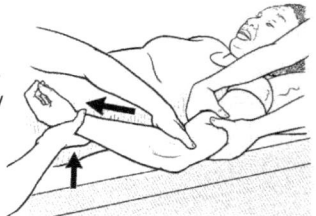

Step 3:

Now push straight down on upper arm as you bend the elbow the rest of the way. You should feel a "clunk." Splint the elbow to prevent it from slipping out of the joint again.

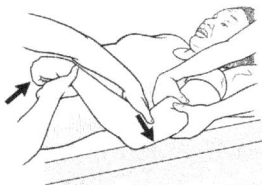

Important

If there is a lot of resistance, stop! You may break the bone. Splint the elbow like this and get medical help.

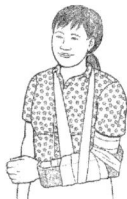

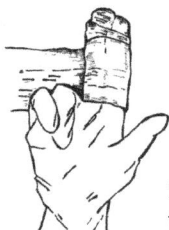

Dislocated finger

Firmly pull a dislocated finger out, and then push the base of the bone into place to set it.

Splint the dislocated finger to the next finger.

Sprains and strains: the twisting or tearing of muscles and ligaments

SIGNS
- Swelling
- Pain
- Bruising or redness

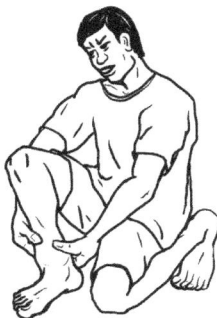

TREATMENT

- **Rest**: do not put weight on the injured part. Using a sling or crutches can help.
- **Ice**: for about 30 minutes every 2 to 4 hours. Less often after a few days.
- **Compress**: wrap firmly with a bandage.
- **Elevate**: raise the injured part using a pillow or folded blankets. Elevate all the time at first, and every few hours after a few days.

These measures will lessen pain and swelling. If started right away and continued, they will help the injured part heal more quickly and with fewer lasting problems.

Keep pressure and weight off the injury. Minor sprains and strains usually take 1 to 2 weeks to heal.

How to wrap a bandage

Start near the toes or fingers.

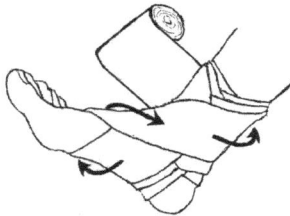

Wrap firmly, but not so tight that toes or fingers get cold or lose feeling.

Bruises

A bruise means that the tissue under the skin has been damaged and some blood is leaking out of the blood vessels. Bruises can hurt a lot and cause concern to the person, but they are usually not a problem. Treat a bruise the same way you would a sprain or strain: with rest, ice, compression, and elevation.

A bruise on the head or abdomen may be a sign of a more serious problem. See what to do if the person recently suffered a hard blow to the head (page 33) or was struck in the abdomen (page 37).

If you notice someone getting bruises often, or with several bruises at different stages of healing, it may be a sign of abuse. Gently try to find out if they are in danger and need help.

Rape and Sexual Violence

Sexual violence is when someone forces another person into any sexual activity. There are many forms of sexual violence including rape, sexual assault, sexual harassment, and stalking. Sexual violence can happen to anyone, but happens most often to women and girls. A victim of rape or sexual assault often knows their attacker—they may be a family member, date, classmate, friend, boyfriend, or husband. For more on rape and sexual violence, see Chapter 19 in Hesperian's *Where Women Have No Doctor*.

A person who has been raped or sexually assaulted will need first aid to treat any injuries and medicines to prevent pregnancy and sexually transmitted infections (STIs). Emotional support is also very important. Treat people who have been raped with kindness and understanding; do not blame them.

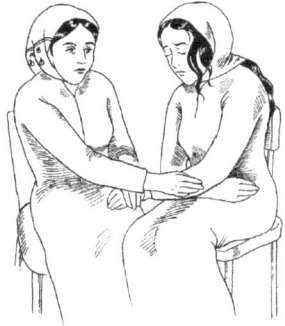

Someone who was raped may find it difficult for you to look at or touch their body, so explain what you will be doing as you begin each step of your examination or treatment. Ask for permission each time before touching.

Rape and sexual assault can cause pregnancy. Emergency contraception (using special pills, certain IUDs, or some types of birth control pills) can prevent pregnancy when used within 5 days of sex.

Mark down all the injuries that you find and, if you have permission, take photographs. These can help you see how injuries are healing when you follow up. They can also be used as proof that violence or a crime took place.

If the anus or genitals have tears, cuts, or bruises, these will be painful. Give paracetamol (acetaminophen) or ibuprofen. If there is a lot of bleeding in the anus or vagina, show how to use pressure to stop it, in case bleeding starts again later.

For small cuts and tears, soak in warm water 3 times a day. Pouring water over the genitals while passing urine may help reduce discomfort. Larger cuts or tears may need to be sutured.

Look for injuries to other areas of the body as well, and see other parts of this guide to treat specific problems. A record of the physical exam and any injuries is necessary if the case is reported to the police, even if a decision to go to the police is not made until much later.

Follow up with the person after a few days to see how they are doing emotionally and physically. Check cuts or tears for signs of infection. Bladder infections are especially common for women after forced or violent sex. Pain or a burning sensation while passing urine, and feeling like you need to pass urine very often, are common signs of bladder infection.

Burns

Minor burns

A minor burn is small, does not form blisters, does not affect the face, hands, feet, genitals or any joints, and is the only injury a person has sustained. To lessen pain and damage, put the burned area in clean cool water (not ice or ice water) right away for no longer than 20 minutes. Then keep the burn clean and dry and take aspirin, paracetamol (acetaminophen), or ibuprofen for pain (avoid giving aspirin to children). Minor burns should heal by themselves within about 2 weeks.

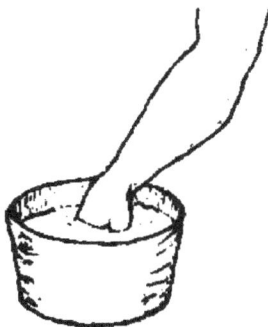

Severe burns

A burn is severe when any of the following is true:
- **The burn is large.** A large burn covers 10% or more of the body. You can estimate how much of the body is burned based on the size of the palm of the hand of the burned person. The size of one palm is about 1% of their body surface. 10 palms is about 10%.
- **The burn affects a joint, the face, the hands, the feet, or the genitals.** These can scar and cause disabilities.
- **The burn is combined with other injuries.**
- **The burn is deep.** Deep burns affect many layers of skin. It is often difficult to tell how deep a burn is right after it has happened.
- **The burn is on a child.** Children have much more difficulty recovering from burns and whenever possible should be cared for in hospitals equipped to treat burns.

TREATMENT

To prevent infection, wash a severe burn with water that has been boiled and cooled, and add povidone iodine if you can (mix 4 parts boiled/cooled water with 1 part povidone iodine). Scrub gently so the burn does not bleed and rinse with more boiled and cooled water. Then dry the burn by blotting with sterile gauze or sterilized cloth. Wearing sterile gloves, put one of the following directly on the burn to kill germs:

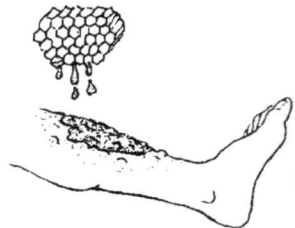

- silver sulfadiazine: Use a thin layer. Do not use for burns on eyelids or lips, or to burns on children younger than 2 months old.

- honey: Use a thin layer.

- sugar: Pour granulated sugar to cover the burn. Throw away any sugar that does not stick to the burn.

Then gently cover the burn with sterile gauze or sterilized cloth and secure this with tape or bandages. If the burn is on an arm or leg, keep the limb elevated to lessen swelling.

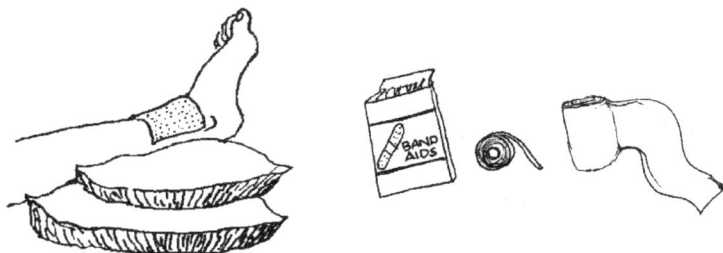

Clean the burn, reapply the antimicrobial agent, and change the covering once each day. Burns are extremely painful. As needed, give strong pain medicine such as morphine (page 123). Always give pain medicine before cleaning or changing a dressing on a serious burn. As burns heal they can start to itch. An antihistamine can provide some relief (pages 110 to 111).

Never put ice, grease, fat, hides, coffee, herbs, or feces on a burn. If signs of infection appear—pus, bad smell, fever, or swollen lymph nodes—put an antibiotic ointment such as Polysporin on the burn and get medical attention as soon as possible. The person needs surgery to clean the wound and intravenous antibiotics to treat the infection.

SPECIAL PRECAUTIONS FOR VERY SERIOUS BURNS

• A person with a large or deep burn can easily become dehydrated because body fluids are lost as they ooze from the burn. Give intravenous (IV) fluids if you can. Otherwise, give large quantities of rehydration drink to someone who is alert and able to swallow. Watch for danger signs of shock (page 17) that can come from dehydration.

• When someone is badly burned between their fingers, in their armpit, or at other joints, put gauze pads with petroleum jelly between the burned surfaces to prevent them from scarring together as they heal.

• Plenty of nutritious food, including extra protein, is needed to heal a burn. While healing, help the person eat at least 4 meals each day that have protein (such as chicken, other meats, eggs, milk, fish, beans, and nuts), as well as snacks

• Burned parts of the body may become stiff and immobile as they heal and scar tissue forms, especially if the burn is on a joint. Help the person gently move the burned part of their body immediately after the injury, and do this 2 to 3 times each day until the burned skin no longer tightens and shrinks (usually many months to years after a burn).

As with any serious injury, get help if the person gets worse or you cannot provide needed care.

Electric shock

Electric shock can cause burns
and stop the heart.

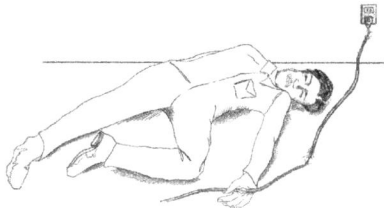

First cut the power or use a non-metal tool
to move the wire. Then move the person.
This protects you from getting shocked too.

1. **If a person is being
   shocked**: Do not touch the
   person. The electricity can
   pass through his body and
   shock anyone who touches
   him. First, unplug or turn
   off the machine or tool
   causing the shock. If you cannot turn off the power, use dry
   clothing, rope, or a piece of wood, such as a broom handle,
   as a tool to separate the victim from the power source. Do
   not use anything wet or made of metal. If the person is
   lying in water, use the wood or cloth to drag him out, and
   do not step in the water yourself! Then you can move the
   person away from the source of electricity.

2. Electric shock can cause breathing to stop. Start rescue
   breathing (pages 10 to 11).

3. If there is no heartbeat try to start the heart by giving chest
   compressions—press hard and fast on the middle of the
   chest (pages 12 to 13). It may take a long time. Keep trying.

4. If the person is breathing and her heart is beating, look for
   signs of burns. As with a gunshot wound, there should be
   both an entry and exit burn.

5. Check for other injuries. Mental confusion, nerve damage
   (problems with feeling or movement), hearing loss, or
   circulation problems can all arise. If the person fell, he may
   have a head injury, broken bones, or bleeding.

If the shock was low-voltage, and the person has no sign of problems after a few hours, he will likely be OK. If the shock was high-voltage or from lightening, or if the person has lingering problems, be more cautious. Burns inside the body can be much more severe than burns on the skin where the electricity entered and left the body. IV fluids and other remedies may be needed. It may take days or weeks to know the real damage.

Chemical Burns

Protect yourself first: Wear long sleeves and gloves or bags over your hands. Cover your mouth with a handkerchief. Wash yourself and your clothing thoroughly after helping anyone who has been exposed to chemicals.

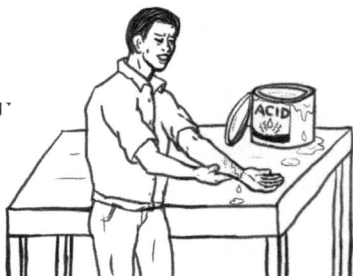

The best way to prevent damage from chemical burns is to **get the chemical off as fast as possible.**

1. Take off clothing and jewelry near the burn.
2. If the chemical is sticky, quickly scrape it off with a flat stick, the side of a knife, or something else stiff.

3. Once you have scraped off all the chemical you can, **rinse the area with lots and lots of water.** Water can cause some chemicals to start burning, so be sure you have first removed as much of the chemical as possible. For an oily chemical, use soap and water. Use a hose or tap if you have one. If the face is affected, wash it first. Especially clean out any cuts or openings in the skin. The faster you start washing and the longer you wash, the better the skin can survive.

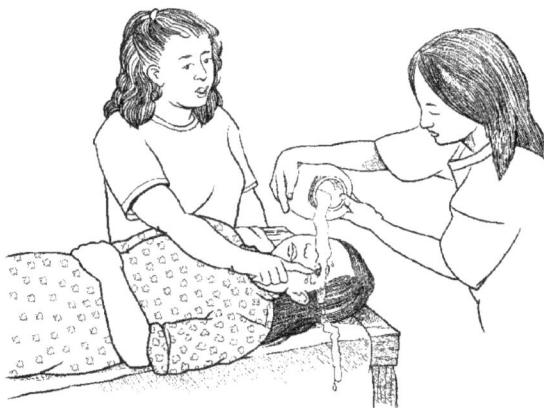

If the chemical got into an eye, pour the water from the inside of the eye (near the nose) toward the outside of the eye (near the ear).

After you have cleaned all the chemical off the person, treat the chemical burn as you would any other burn (page 58).

Wash or discard all clothes that have come into contact with the chemicals, as they can also cause damage.

60

Police Weapons

Be careful: people helping victims of police violence often become targets of more police violence themselves. Try to get the injured person and yourself out of immediate danger.

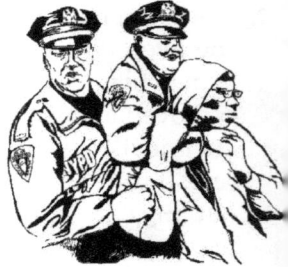

Pepper spray and tear gas

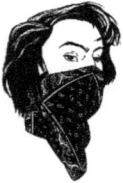

Move away from where tear gas or pepper spray is being used, the effect will wear off. Tear gas wears off quickly, pepper spray can last an hour or more.

A water or vinegar-soaked bandana over the mouth and nose gives a little protection. Make a face shield out of a clear plastic bottle to protect your eyes in case chemicals are sprayed directly at you.

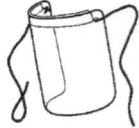

Do not touch tear gas canisters with your hands. They are hot and will burn you if you pick them up right away.

1. **Watch breathing.** Pepper spray can cause severe breathing problems, especially in people with asthma. This can be very frightening. Help the person stay calm.

2. **Flush eyes** with lots of water. Pour the water from the inside of the eye (near the nose) toward the outside of the eye (near the ear).

3. **Remove clothes** that have spray on them once you are in a safe place and will not be exposed to any more spray or chemicals.

4. **Clean the skin, one area at a time (or just wait for the spray to wear off):** soak a cloth with mineral or vegetable oil. Wipe off one area of skin using this oiled cloth.

Then quickly remove the oil with another cloth wet with alcohol. If the oil is left on for more than 30 seconds, it will mix with the chemical and burn the skin. If you do not have oil and alcohol, just use a lot of water. Or just wait. With time, the pain will go away.

Other police weapons

Rubber bullets, tear gas canisters, water cannons, and batons are all used to cause bleeding, broken bones, or injuries inside the body. Injuries to the eye and head can be severe. Examine the person head to toe. Watch for signs of internal bleeding or shock: feeling faint, pale skin, dropping blood pressure, and a weak, fast pulse.

Mental Health Emergency

When someone's thinking and perceptions make them want to hurt themselves or others, this is an emergency and they need help quickly. As with any other emergency, first try to check breathing, stop any bleeding, and check for other physical injuries. Then reassuring, calming, and comforting a person having a mental health emergency can save lives.

If someone says he wants to hurt himself or others, believe him.

If the person is dangerous to others, it is often easier to move other people away than to move him. You may need help to make him and the area around him safe. And look out for your own safety as well.

If he says he wants to hurt or kill himself, the first thing he needs is someone to listen calmly. Asking gentle questions can help interrupt his thoughts and get him the support he needs.

If someone says they plan to hurt themselves or someone else, or you suspect they do:

- **Show concern** but not alarm.

- **Ask directly**, for example, "Are you having thoughts of ending your life?" or "Are you thinking about harming someone else?"

- **People in crisis may feel undecided about suicide.** Focus on supporting the part of the person that wants to live, while not ignoring or downplaying the part of them that wants to die.

- **Suicide crises are often time-limited.** Your goal is to get the person the help they need to get through the crisis and into a different emotional state where they can get longer-term help.

- **Be collaborative and honest.** Say, for example, "I think it is important for you to connect with someone at the clinic about how you are feeling and what might help. Would you be willing to ride over there with me?"

- **You do not have to help the person all by yourself.** Talk with them for a while about what they are experiencing, and then say, "I am worried about your safety and I feel it is important for others who care about you to know you are feeling this way. Can we call your sister to help us think this through?" Or "I am worried about your safety and I would like us to call a hotline together so someone with more experience can help."

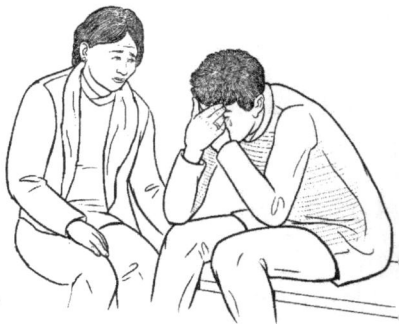

Poison

For most poisons: quickly flush the poison out by drinking **large amounts of water. Taking activated charcoal** (page 115) will also help. If you know the specific poison, see the chart on pages 64 to 67 for information on what to do.

Do not give water, charcoal, or anything else to swallow to someone who cannot breathe well or is losing consciousness. Maintaining breathing is always most important.

Vomiting is not usually helpful for poisoning, and it can be dangerous. Someone who has swallowed corrosive chemicals like acids or lye, or gasoline, kerosene, or turpentine, or who is having trouble breathing should never try to vomit up the poison.

If you do try to vomit, do so as soon as possible, within the first few hours. To encourage vomiting, touch the back of the throat with a finger or swallow a spoonful of salt.

PREVENTION

Poisoning is preventable. Label all poisons and medicines clearly. Keep them out of the reach of children in high or locked cabinets. Never use empty poison containers for food or drink even if you clean them first. Likewise never put poisons in bottles or containers made to be used for food or drink.

Keep all poisons out of the reach of

Poison is a common method people use to kill or harm themselves. Locking away poisons, guns, and other potentially deadly materials is a surprisingly effective way to prevent suicide deaths. For more on how to help someone who wants to kill himself, see "Mental Health Emergency," page 61.

CHEMICAL POISONING

Types of chemicals	⚠ Signs of poisoning

Corrosives:

- Ammonia
- Batteries
- Acids
- Drain cleaner
- Caustic soda
- Lye

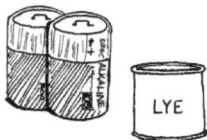

Acids or bases. These chemicals burn the inside of the body.

- Extra saliva.
- Pain in mouth, throat, chest, stomach, or back.
- Vomiting.
- Difficulty swallowing.

Hydrocarbons:

- Gasoline
- Carbolic acid
- Turpentine
- Camphor
- Paint thinner
- Pine oil
- Kerosene
- Phenol

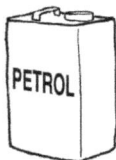

These are most dangerous if breathed into the lungs.

- Difficulty breathing.
- Coughing, choking, gagging.
- Fever.
- Seizures or loss of consciousness (passing out).
- The breath may smell like the poison.

Cyanide:

Used in: mining, factory work, animal hide hair removal (tanning), rat poison.

Can be breathed in or swallowed from contaminated food or water.

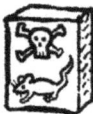

Indoor fires can cause you to breathe cyanide that was in the burning materials. You may smell bitter almond in smoke that has cyanide in it.

- Breathing problems.
- Headache, confusion, and seizures.
- There can be long lasting injury to the brain.

✚ What to do

- **Do not try to vomit.**
- Activated charcoal is of little use.
- Give as much water as you can.
- Get help.

- **Do not try to vomit.**
- Do not give activated charcoal.
- Give a lot of water.
- Wash hydrocarbons off skin and hair and take off any contaminated clothes.
- Give help with breathing if needed (pages 10 to 11) and watch the person's breathing for 2 days.
- Get help.

- **Do not try to vomit.**
- Watch for breathing problems and try to restart the heart if it stops (pages 12 to 13).
- Do not give rescue breathing without a mask.
- Give lots of water.
- Can be treated with sodium nitrite followed by sodium thiosulfate (pages 118 to 119).

CHEMICAL POISONING

Types of chemicals	⚠ Signs of poisoning

Organophosphates and carbamate.

Found in certain pesticides including:

- malathion
- parathion

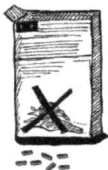

These chemicals can stop breathing or cause other whole-body problems.

- Slowing pulse, muscle weakness, breathing problems.
- Runny nose, crying, drooling.
- Seizures.
- The breath may smell like fuel or garlic.
- Life-threatening problems can happen days after this poison is taken, and long-term nerve problems can happen weeks after.

Herbicides:

- Paraquat (Gramoxone, Cyclone, Herbikill, Dextrone, and many other brand names)
- Glyphosate (Roundup, Touchdown, other brand names)

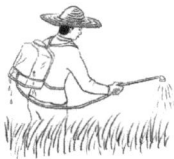

Can be absorbed through the skin, by breathing it in, or most dangerously, by swallowing.

- Breathing problems (can happen days after).
- Mouth pain.
- Red or brown urine, or little or no urine (a sign that the kidney is failing—very dangerous).
- Large quantities can cause burns in the mouth and throat, stomach pain, and breathing problems.

✚ What to do

- Watch for breathing problems and give rescue breathing if needed.

- Atropine is an antidote (page 116).

- Give activated charcoal if it has been less than 1 hour since the poisoning (page 115).

- Wash the skin right away and throw out contaminated clothes.

- Treat seizures with diazepam (page 125).

- Watch for breathing problems and give rescue breathing if needed.
- Give activated charcoal (page 115).
- Get help.

POISONING WITH MEDICINES AND OTHER DRUGS

Types of Drugs	⚠ Signs of overdose

Iron:

- Ferrous sulfate
- Ferrous gluconate
- Prenatal vitamins
- Multivitamin pills or syrups

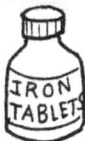

An overdose damages the stomach and intestines.

- Pain, vomit or bloody vomit, diarrhea, confusion.
- Shock immediately or up to 2 days later.

Paracetamol:

- Acetaminophen (Panadol, Tylenol, Crocin, and other brand names)
- Many combination cold medicines and pain medicines (read the label)

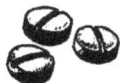

An overdose is poisonous to the liver.

- Nausea, sweating, pale skin, tiredness.
- Later there may be liver pain (right upper belly), jaundice, confusion, or bloody urine.

Opioid medicines:

- Morphine
- Heroin
- Methadone
- Opium
- Oxycodone
- Other strong pain medicines

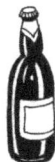

An overdose can cause the person to stop breathing.

- Slow thinking, slow reactions, slow, shallow, or stopped breathing.

Alcohol

An overdose can cause the person to stop breathing.

- Vomiting.
- Confusion.
- Seizures.
- Slow or irregular breathing.
- Loss of consciousness. Confusion, changes in consciousness, irregular breathing, and feeling or looking ill could also be signs of a diabetic emergency (page 70).

✚ What to do

- Immediate vomiting may help.
- Give lots and lots of water.
- Activated charcoal is not helpful.
- Deferoxamine is an antidote (page 117).
- Watch for breathing problems.

- If you can get the person to vomit right away it may be of some help.
- Give activated charcoal (page 115) and lots of water.
- Acetylcysteine is an antidote (page 117).

- If the person is breathing fewer than 12 breaths a minute give rescue breathing (pages 10 to 11).
- Naloxone is an antidote (page 118).
- Do not let the person drink or swallow until

- Monitor the person's breathing and give rescue breathing if necessary.
- Turn him on his side to prevent choking if he vomits.
- Keep the person warm.
- If the person is able to drink, give Rehydration Drink (page 81).

Diabetic Emergencies

Diabetes is a disease that affects the body's ability to process sugars in food. Someone with diabetes can suddenly become ill if he has too much, or too little, sugar in his blood.

If you know someone is having an emergency due to diabetes but you are not sure if the problem is from low blood sugar or high blood sugar, treat as if he has low blood sugar (give a small amount of sugar), and then take him to get medical help.

Low blood sugar (hypoglycemia)

This condition can only happen to a person treating his diabetes with medicines. A person's blood sugar can drop too low if he is taking insulin or another diabetes medication and if he takes too much medicine, does not eat enough food, does too much physical activity, waits too long between meals, or drinks alcohol.

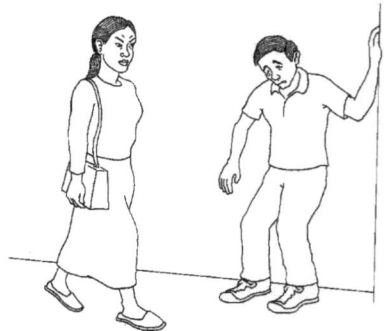

Low blood sugar can look a lot like the person is drunk and can be overlooked as being a real emergency.

Someone with low blood sugar may become clumsy, confused, nervous, or irritable. He may sweat or tremble. When that happens, he must eat. If he does not, his condition will worsen and will develop these danger signs:

DANGER SIGNS
- Trouble walking or feeling weak
- Trouble seeing clearly
- Confusion or acting in a strange way (you may mistake him for being drunk)
- Losing consciousness
- Seizure

TREATMENT

If he is conscious, quickly give him sugar: fruit juice, soda, candy, or a glass of water with several spoons of sugar in it will all work. He should eat a full meal soon after as well. If he is still confused or does not begin to feel better 15 minutes after you have given sugar, get help.

If he is unconscious, place a pinch of sugar or honey under his tongue. Keep giving small amounts. It takes time for the body to absorb sugar. When he wakes up you can give him more.

High blood sugar (hyperglycemia)

A person with diabetes can have too much sugar in his blood if he eats too much food, is less active than usual, has a serious illness or infection, does not take his diabetes medicine, or gets dehydrated. This can happen to a person even if he does not yet know he has diabetes. Get help for these signs:

SIGNS
- Feeling thirsty and drinking a lot
- Frequent urination
- Blurry vision
- Weight loss
- Nausea and vomiting
- Abdominal pain

If not treated, high blood sugar can be very dangerous and can lead to a coma or even death. You can save a person's life by getting help for these more dangerous signs:

DANGER SIGNS
- Fast heart rate
- Fruity odor on breath
- Dry skin
- Low blood pressure
- Confusion
- Fast, deep breathing
- Loss of consciousness

TREATMENT
Take him immediately to a medical center. If he is conscious, give him plenty of water to drink. Give a little at a time.

If you are certain he has high blood sugar and know his insulin dose, give a small amount of insulin on the way to help. But if you are not certain, do not give insulin. Giving someone insulin when they have low blood sugar can kill them.

Seizures, Convulsions

Seizures are sudden, usually brief, periods of change in consciousness or mental state. Someone having a seizure may lose consciousness or have convulsions (jerking movements). Or they may have few or no physical signs and just be "absent."

Seizures can be caused by high fever, meningitis, dehydration, a head injury, malaria, or poisoning, among other reasons. If none of these seem likely, a single seizure may not be a reason for concern (although it can be very frightening to watch).

Seizures that repeat over a long period of time are often from epilepsy, a chronic condition that can be controlled with medicines. See a health worker.

TREATMENT

During a seizure, clear the space around the person so she is not injured. Turn her on her side so she does not choke if she vomits. **Do not hold a seizing person down or put anything in her mouth or between her teeth. Get medical help.**

If the seizure lasts more than 5 minutes, put liquid diazepam in the anus using a syringe without a needle. Do not give more than the recommended dose and do not give more than 2 doses (page 125).

For seizure from **dehydration:** after the seizure is over, give plenty of fluids, like water and Rehydration Drink (page 81).

For seizure from **meningitis:** when the seizure is over, take the person to the hospital right away. She will need a combination of specific antibiotics and other emergency medical help.

For seizure from **malaria:** treat the malaria as soon as possible with the medicines used in your region, usually ACT (artemisinin-based combination therapy). Seizures and convulsions can be a sign of severe malaria, which can cause death if not treated quickly.

The spasms caused by **tetanus** can be mistaken for seizures. The jaw shuts tightly (lockjaw) and the body suddenly bends back. Learn to recognize early signs of tetanus,
see page 29.

After a seizure, the person may be confused or tired. Comfort her.

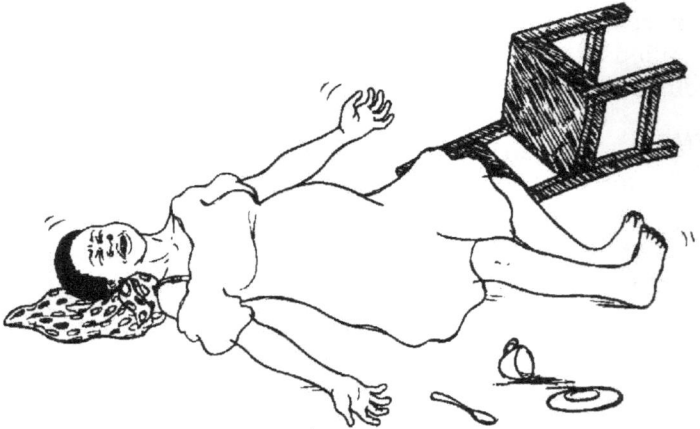

Stings and Bites

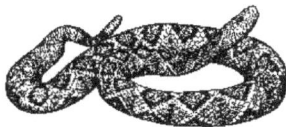

Most bites and stings are painful but not dangerous, and even deadly creatures do not usually inject enough venom to kill. Stay calm and watch the bitten part. If there are no problems or if problems improve after a few hours (depending on the creature) there is likely nothing to worry about. Because children are small, the venom can affect them and do more harm, so they may need more attention.

Do not cut open a bite or sting or try to suck out the poison. Also, tourniquets will not stop the spread of poisons from stings or bites, but will cause serious harm.

Snake bites

1. Move away from the snake. Some snakes can still bite for a few minutes even after they are dead.
2. Remove jewelry or clothes near the bite because the body may swell.
3. Keep the bitten part of the body below the heart. **Then keep that body part still** by putting on a splint or sling. Using the muscles spreads the poison.
4. Gently clean the wound. Do not rub it.
5. For most snakes, or if you do not know what type it was, watch and wait for a few hours. If there is little or no swelling, pain, or redness, there is no problem. Danger signs include severe swelling or pain, drowsiness, droopy eyelids, dizziness, weakness, nausea, or bleeding from the mouth or nose.

Ask the person to swish water in the mouth and spit in a light-colored bowl. If the spit is pink or visibly bloody, the gums are bleeding. This is a danger sign.

76

For these snakes, wrap the bitten area tightly:

- Coral snakes
- Mambas
- South American rattlesnakes
- Sea snakes
- Most cobras—the ones that cause damage throughout the whole body

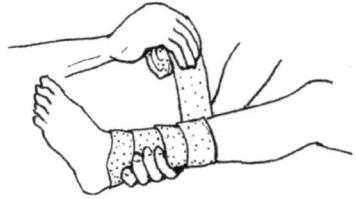

Wrap tight—to stop the spread of poison, but not so tight that you cut off blood flow.

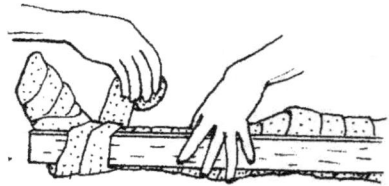

Use a splint to keep the limb from moving.

Most vipers and some cobras harm the area near where they bite but do not cause problems throughout the rest of the body. For these snakes, do not wrap the bite.

For many **poisonous snakes** there is an antivenom that can help. If you can get to medical help, describe the snake as well as you can so the right antivenom is used. If possible, stock your medicine kit with snake antivenom for the snakes common in your area before emergencies happen.

For spitting cobra venom in the eye: flush with a lot of water. If you have no water, milk or beer can be used. Do not use strong irritating chemicals.

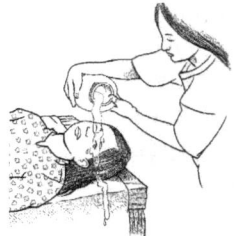

Pythons and boas are not poisonous, but their bites can cause severe skin infections. Watch the wound and if there are signs of infection—increasing redness, heat, pain, swelling, bad smell, or pus—treat it as an infected wound (pages 27 to 28). Occasionally these snakes cause crush injuries by squeezing a person.

If the bite mark shows fangs, the snake is venomous. If there are no fang marks, it is less likely that the snake is poisonous, but it still could be.

Spiders and scorpions

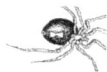

Although they may hurt a lot, most spider bites and scorpion stings do not cause serious or lasting harm. Keep the bitten part still and use ice or cold water to relieve pain. Do not cut open the bite or use a tourniquet or bandage. Heat does not help, but keeping still does.

If you know the spider or scorpion is a deadly variety, or, if after the bite or sting there are signs of problems such as: stomachache, itching, sweating, and difficulty breathing, then get medical help. There may be an antivenom.

For Black Widow spider bites or scorpion stings, you can give diazepam on the way to medical help to prevent muscle spasms and calm the person (pages 124 to 125).

Bees and wasps

After a sting, check if a stinger was left in the skin and remove it as soon as possible. The area around the sting may get red, swollen, and painful. Putting a paste made with baking soda and water, or something cold on the stung area, will help with the swelling and pain.

Severe allergy to bee or wasp stings is rare, but can be deadly. See pages 79 to 80 for signs and treatment of severe allergy.

Ticks

A bite from a tick can spread many dangerous infections. Check your body well after walking where ticks are common. To remove a tick with tweezers, grasp the tick as close as possible to where its mouth is stuck to the skin. Pull it out gently but firmly so that its head does not remain under the skin. Burn the removed tick with a match or kill it with alcohol, but try not to touch it.

Fish and jellyfish

Get away from jellyfish and scrape off any tentacles. Use seawater to wash. For stinging fish, remove any spines with tweezers or pliers.

Immerse the limb in hot water for 20 minutes to relieve pain, but make sure it is not burning hot. This may work better for stinging fish than for jellies.

There are many local remedies but they do not work for all fish or jellyfish. For example, box jellyfish (sea wasp) stings are helped by washing with vinegar. But vinegar makes the stings of other jellyfish worse. Papaya or meat tenderizer is a well-known home remedy for jellyfish stings but it does not seem to work for all jellyfish and sometimes makes the pain worse.

Allow the person to use and move their limbs—unlike with snake and spider bites, keeping still does not help. Get medical help if there are problems breathing or other signs get worse.

Allergy: Mild or Severe (Anaphylaxis)

Mild allergies are caused by dust, pollen, insect bites, or certain foods, chemicals, or medicines. These are usually treatable with antihistamines (pages 110 to 111).

SIGNS OF A MILD ALLERGY (ALLERGIC REACTION)

Itching, swollen, red eyes

Rash or redness

Sneezing

If there is an insect bite, it may swell

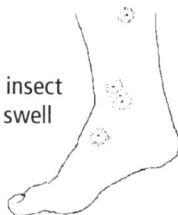

A severe allergy is much more dangerous and can quickly stop someone's breathing. Common causes include antibiotics (especially penicillins), antitoxins made from horse serum, and the sting of wasps or bees.

SIGNS OF A SEVERE ALLERGY (ALLERGIC SHOCK, ANAPHYLAXIS)

- Flushing, itching, or rash
- Swollen lips, mouth, or throat
- Difficulty breathing or swallowing
- Swollen hands or feet
- Nausea or stomachache

The most common signs are rash and breathing problems.

If the person cannot swallow or is having trouble breathing, **give epinephrine right away** (pages 112 to 113). Have this ready in a medicine kit **before** emergencies happen. Or include a pre-loaded epinephrine injection, called an *Epipen* in many places.

Inject epinephrine in the thigh muscle, here:

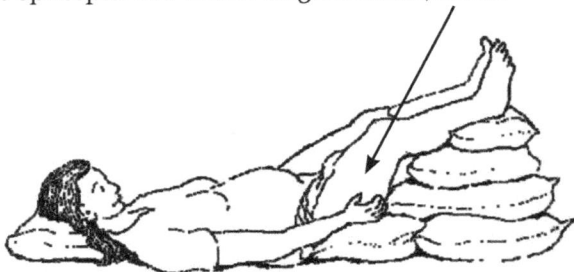

Elevate the feet above the heart

For breathing problems you can also give salbutamol (page 113). To treat symptoms such as itch and rash, you can give an antihistamine (pages 110 to 111).

In most cases, if you ever have an allergic reaction to a medicine, food, bee sting, or something else, you should avoid it forever after. The second time you are exposed you can expect an even worse reaction.

Heat Emergencies

Heat cramps and heat exhaustion (heat sickness)

Working hard in hot conditions can cause painful cramps in the legs, arms, or stomach. This is probably caused by losing too much salt from sweating. Gently stretch out cramps, by moving the feet, or slowly walking.

Treat heat exhaustion (heat sickness) as soon as signs appear. If not treated, heat exhaustion can worsen into heat stroke.

SIGNS
- Extreme thirst.
- Weakness.
- Headache.
- Nausea or abdominal cramps.
- The skin is usually sweaty and may be cool and pale.
- There may be a prickly feeling on the skin or a rash.

TREATMENT
- Rest in a cool place. Take off extra clothes.
- Give Rehydration Drink—mix ½ teaspoon salt and 8 teaspoons of sugar or cooked cereal in 1 liter water.
- Give plenty of other cool liquids too.

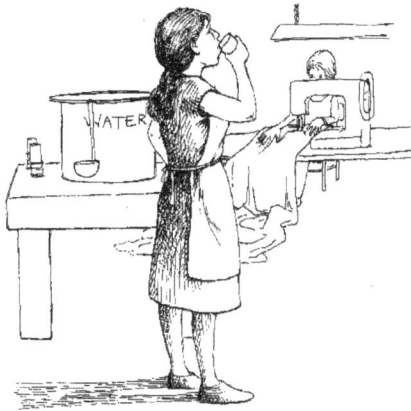

Heat stroke

Heat stroke is a very dangerous condition that is caused by being too hot for too long. Left untreated, it can kill.

SIGNS

- Fast pulse and fast breathing
- Skin flushed (red), warm, dry, or clammy
- Vomiting or diarrhea
- Confusion
- Passing out or seizures
- High fever, greater than 40°C (104°F)

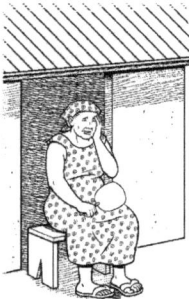

Heat stroke happens to people who are not able to recover quickly from getting too hot. People who are very young or very old, who are pregnant, who have certain medical conditions like heart disease or diabetes, or who drink large amounts of alcohol are most likely to develop heat stroke during hot weather.

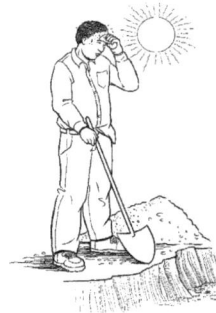

Heat stroke can also happen to a healthy young adult who has worked or exercised too long in the heat. These people tend to be sweaty instead of having dry skin.

TREATMENT

Cool the person as fast as possible: move to the shade. Take off extra clothes. Fan the person and wipe them with cool, wet cloths all over the body. Put ice packs or cold cloths on the neck, armpits, and groin. An otherwise healthy person can be dunked in a bath of ice-cold water, but this is dangerous for an old person or someone who is already ill.

When the person is alert, give Rehydration Drink (page 81). Or give a lot of any cool drink. But be careful the person does not choke: breathing problems are common with heat stroke.

Someone with heat stroke can get worse quickly so if possible it is best to get medical help.

PREVENTION

To prevent heat-related problems outside, wear light-colored clothing and shade the face and back of the neck with a hat. Indoor work spaces should have enough air flow and fans. Take regular breaks and drink lots of liquids. Avoid or limit drinking beer and other alcohol while working or playing sports in the heat because alcohol causes dehydration.

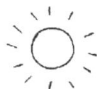

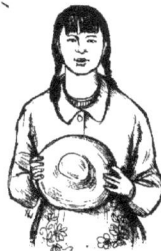

Sunburns

Problems with sunburn are often more serious for people with light skin color. The skin becomes red, painful, and hot, and in severe cases it will blister and swell. Blisters from sunburn, as from other burns, can get easily infected. A single sunburn is not dangerous, but many sunburns over time can lead to skin cancer.

A sunburn will heal on its own after a few days. Aloe or a mild pain medicine can help. There may be some local treatments in your area that cool and relieve the skin.

PREVENTION
Wear a hat and clothing that covers the skin when the sun is strong. Sunscreen lotion that is rubbed into the skin before going into the sun can also help prevent sunburn.

Cold Emergencies

Hypothermia (getting too cold)

Being too cold for too long can be deadly. It can quickly cause confusion, affect judgment, and make it harder to think clearly about how to get warm.

SIGNS
- Shivering
- Fast breathing and heart rate
- Difficulty speaking clearly, clumsiness
- Confusion
- Having to urinate more

As hypothermia gets worse, the pulse and breathing may slow down. The person may sit down, stop shivering, and in her confusion may start to take off clothes. Eventually she can pass out or die.

TREATMENT

Give rescue breathing if needed (pages 10 to 11). A very cold person can recover after a long time of not breathing, so you may need to give rescue breathing for an hour or more.

- Get somewhere warm and dry.
- Remove wet clothes.
- Cover in warm, dry blankets. Be sure to cover head, hands, and feet.

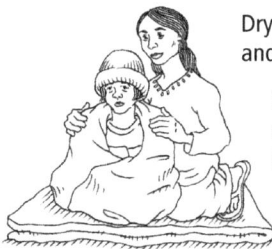

Dry clothes, blankets, and a hat

Body heat (or hot stones, or hot water bottles)

Warm, sweet drinks

- Do all you can to keep the person warm. Cuddle up close to the person, heat stones and then wrap them in cloth, or use hot water bottles to warm the person. But beware of burning the skin.

Folded blankets or cardboard protect from the cold ground

If the person can sit up and hold a cup, give warm drinks. Do not give alcoholic drinks. While they may feel "hot" in your throat or stomach, alcoholic drinks cause the body to lose heat. Also give food. Candy and sweets are especially helpful. Give a meal soon after. Encourage the person to drink plenty of water.

If the person has severe hypothermia—a body temperature of 32°C (90°F) or less, is unconscious, not shivering anymore—be as gentle as you can while quickly transporting her to help.

Frostbite (frozen body parts)

Toes, fingers, ears, and other body parts can freeze. Eventually they "die," turning black. If you act fast at the first signs of frostbite, you can save these body parts that otherwise might need to be cut off.

SIGNS

- Skin cold, waxy, pale, splotchy
- Tingling, numbness, or pain
- The body part may be frozen hard

Light, mild frostbite turns the skin red. A few days later it peels. If it is a bit deeper, frostbite leaves the skin feeling hard, but soft underneath. Blisters may form the next day. When the muscle freezes, the frostbite is deep. The area is hard. It may blister only at the edges, or not at all. The blisters may fill with blood.

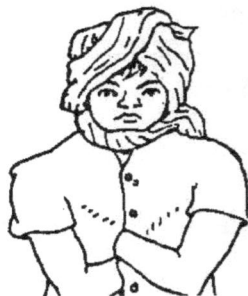

TREATMENT

Get out of the cold and quickly warm the frozen part. For fingers, the easiest thing is for the person to hold her hands in her own armpits or between her thighs. Or wrap the frozen parts in warm, dry cloths. Keep the frozen area still and try not to walk on frostbitten feet.

For deeper frostbite, fill a basin with warm (not hot) water. If you have a thermometer, try for 39°C (102°F). Soak the frozen part in the water. Check the water first to prevent burns. **Do not rub.**

The frozen part should thaw within 45 minutes. As it warms, it will hurt. Give pain medicine (page 119). Do not let it become frozen again.

It is better to let the area stay frozen than to thaw it and let it freeze again.

As frostbite heals over the coming days and weeks, treat it as you would a burn (pages 53 to 56).

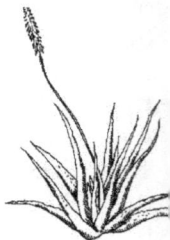

Aloe helps heal frostbite and burns

Medicines
Antibiotics Fight Infection

Antibiotics are medicines that fight infections caused by bacteria. They do not help against infections from a virus such as chicken pox, rubella, flu, or the common cold. Not all antibiotics will fight all infections from bacteria.

Antibiotics that share the same chemical make-up are said to be from the same family. It is important to know about the families of antibiotics for two reasons:

1. Antibiotics from the same family can often treat the same problems.

2. If you are allergic to one antibiotic in a family, it is likely you will be allergic to other antibiotics in that family. It is safest for you to take an antibiotic from another family instead.

Antibiotics must be taken for their full course. Stopping before you have finished all the days of treatment, even if you feel better, can make the infection return in a form that is even harder to stop.

The penicillins

Antibiotics in the penicillin family are useful against many infections. Penicillins are safe to use during pregnancy and breastfeeding. They are widely available, low cost, and available in oral and injectable forms.

Resistance to penicillins

Certain infections have become resistant to penicillins. This means that penicillins would have cured these infections in the past but no longer work. If an infection does not respond to treatment with a penicillin, try an antibiotic from another family. For example, pneumonia is sometimes resistant to penicillin. Try cotrimoxazole or erythromycin.

Important ⚠ for all kinds of penicillin (including ampicillin and amoxicillin)

Penicillins can cause mild allergic reactions in some people (for example, rash and itching). Often this comes hours or days after taking the medicine and may last for days. Stop taking the medicine immediately and take an antihistamine (pages 110 to 111) to calm the itching. Stomach upset and diarrhea from taking penicillins are not signs of an allergic reaction and, while uncomfortable, are not a reason to stop taking them.

In rare cases, pencillins can cause severe allergic reactions (allergic shock or **anaphylaxis**, page 79) within a few minutes or hours after taking the medicine. This is very dangerous. Epinephrine (adrenaline, page 112) must be injected at once. Always have epinephrine ready when you inject penicillin.

Someone who has had an allergic reaction to a pencillin should not be given any other kind of penicillin, including ampicillin or amoxicillin, by mouth or by injection, ever again. The next time, the allergic reaction will likely be worse and may even cause death. People allergic to penicillin can use antibiotics from other families, such as erythromycin.

Injections

Use injected forms of penicillin only for severe or dangerous infections. Injectable penicillins are more likely to cause severe allergic reactions and other problems, and should be used with caution. Penicillin taken by mouth usually works well.

Ampicillin and Amoxicillin

Ampicillin and amoxicillin are broad-spectrum penicillins, which means they kill many kinds of bacteria. The two are often interchangeable. When you see a recommendation for ampicillin in this book, you can often use amoxicillin in its place if you know the correct dose.

Ampicillin and amoxicillin are very safe and are especially useful for babies and small children.

Side effects

Both these medicines, but especially ampicillin, tend to cause nausea and diarrhea. Avoid giving them to people who already have diarrhea if you can give another antibiotic instead.

These medicines may also cause a rash. If the rash is flat and not itchy, appears several days to weeks after taking ampicillin or amoxicillin, and is not accompanied by other symptoms, then it is likely not a reason for concern.

But if a raised, itchy rash develops within a few hours of taking ampicillin or amoxicilin, this is a sign of a penicillin allergy. Stop giving the medicine right away and do not give the person a penicillin medicine again. Future allergic reactions are likely to be more severe and may even be life-threatening (see "Signs of a severe allergy (allergic shock, anaphylaxis)," page 79). If you cannot tell for sure if the rash is from allergy, it is safest to stop taking the medicine and take an antibiotic from a different family.

Important ⚠

More infections are becoming resistant to ampicillin and amoxicillin. Depending on where you live, they may no longer work against staphylococcus, shigella, or other infections.

How to use

Ampicillin and amoxicillin work well when taken by mouth. Ampicillin can also be given by injection for severe illnesses.

As with other antibiotics, always give these medicines for at least the shorter number of days shown here. If the person still has signs of infection, have her continue taking the same amount every day until all signs of infection have been gone for at least 24 hours. If the person has taken the medicine for the maximum number of days and is still sick, stop giving the antibiotic and get medical help. For people with HIV, always give the medicine for the maximum number of days listed.

The amount of antibiotic to take depends on the age or weight of the person and the severity of the infection. In general, give the smaller amount for a smaller person or a less severe infection, and the larger amount for a larger person or a more severe infection.

AMOXICILLIN (ORAL)

➡ Give 45 to 50 mg per kg each day into muscle, divided into 2 doses a day. If you cannot weigh the person, dose by age:
Under 3 months: give 125 mg, 2 times a day for 7 to 10 days.
3 months to 3 years: give 250 mg, 2 times a day for 7 to 10 days.
4 to 7 years: give 375 mg, 2 times a day for 7 to 10 days.
8 to 12 years: give 500 mg, 2 times a day for 7 to 10 days.
Over 12 years: give 500 to 875 mg, 2 times a day for 7 to 10 days.

AMPICILLIN (ORAL)

➡ Give 50 to 100 mg per kg each day, divided into 4 doses a day. If you cannot weigh the person, dose by age:
Under 1 year: give 100 mg, 4 times a day for 7 days.
1 to 3 years: give 125 mg, 4 times a day for 7 days.
4 to 7 years: give 250 mg, 4 times a day for 7 days.
8 to 12 years: give 375 mg, 4 times a day for 7 days.
Over 12 years: give 500 mg, 4 times a day for 7 days.

AMPICILLIN (INJECTION)

Ampicillin should be injected only for severe illnesses, or when someone is vomiting or cannot swallow.

➡ Inject 100 to 200 mg per kg each day into muscle, divided into 4 doses a day. If you cannot weigh the person, dose by age:
Under 1 year: inject 100 mg, 4 times a day for 7 days.
1 to 5 years: inject 300 mg, 4 times a day for 7 days.
6 to 12 years: inject 625 mg, 4 times a day for 7 days.
Over 12 years: inject 875 mg, 4 times a day for 7 days.

Amoxicillin with clavulanic acid (Amoxicillin-clavulanate potassium)

Amoxicillin with clavulanic acid comes in different strengths of each of the 2 medicines it contains, for example, 500/125 (a 4-to-1 strength because the tablets have 500 mg amoxicillin and 125 mg clavulanic acid) or 875/125 (a 7-to-1 strength). For children, it is best to use the 4-to-1 ratio such as the 500/125 tablet or the liquid medicine where 5 ml contains 125/31.25 or 250/62.5. Often, the dose of amoxicillin with clavulanic acid mentions only the amount of amoxicillin (as we do here).

How to use

Give by mouth with food or milk.

For animal bites

➡ To prevent infection using a 4-to-1 strength such as the 500/125 tablet or a syrup made for children, give 20 mg per kg for 3 to 5 days, divided into 3 doses. If you cannot weigh the person, dose by age:
3 months to 1 year: give 50 mg, 3 times a day for 3 to 5 days.
1 to 5 years: give 125 mg, 3 times a day for 3 to 5 days.
6 to 12 years: give 250 mg, 3 times a day for 3 to 5 days.
Over 12 years: give 250 mg, 3 times a day OR use the 875/125 tablet, 2 times a day for 3 to 5 days.

If the bite is already infected, give the same dose for up to 14 days.

Penicillin by mouth, penicillin V, penicillin VK

Penicillin by mouth (rather than by injection) can be used for mild and moderate infections.

Even if you started with injected penicillin for a severe infection, you can usually switch to penicillin by mouth once the person starts to improve. If improvement does not begin within 2 or 3 days, consider switching to another antibiotic and get medical advice.

How to use

To help the body make better use of the medicine, take penicillin on an empty stomach, at least 1 hour before or 2 hours after meals.

→ Give 25 to 50 mg per kg each day, divided into 4 doses, for 10 days. If you cannot weigh the person, dose by age:

Under 1 year: give 62 mg, 4 times a day for 10 days.

1 to 5 years: give 125 mg, 4 times a day for 10 days.

6 to 12 years: give 125 to 250 mg, 4 times a day for 10 days.

Over 12 years: give 250 to 500 mg, 4 times a day for 10 days.

For animal bites, give the dose above for 3 to 5 days. Also give metronidazole (page 99) OR clindamycin (page 98).

Cloxacillin

Cloxacillin is a form of penicillin, and can sometimes be used for infections that have become resistant to penicillin, such as sores on the skin with pus, and bone infections. If you do not have cloxacillin, dicloxacillin (page 93) can be used instead.

Side effects

Nausea, vomiting, diarrhea, fever, and joint pain.

Important ⚠

- Do not give if the person is allergic to penicillin.

How to use 🖐

For most infections

➡ For young children give 25 to 50 mg per kg, divided into 4 doses a day. For adults give 50 to 100 mg per kg, divided into 4 doses a day. If you cannot weigh the person, dose by age:
Under 2 years: give 75 mg, 4 times a day.
2 to 10 years: give 125 mg, 4 times a day.
Over 10 years: give 250 to 500 mg, 4 times a day.

For knife or gunshot wound, give the dose above for 10 to 14 days. If the wound is dirty or in the abdomen, also give metronidazole (page 99).

For a bone that has broken through the skin (open fracture), give the dose above for 5 to 7 days. If the wound is very dirty, also give metronidazole (page 99).

Dicloxacillin

Dicloxacillin is a form of penicillin, and can sometimes be used for infections that have become resistant to penicillin. If you do not have dicloxacillin, cloxacillin (page 92) can be used instead.

Side effects 🧑

Nausea, stomach pain, loss of appetite.

Important ⚠

- Do not give if the person is allergic to penicillin. Do not give to newborns.
- Stop taking if you begin to have dark urine, gray colored stools, or jaundice (yellow skin and eyes).

How to use

Give with a full glass of water. Give 1 hour before eating, or 2 hours after eating.

➡ For children under 40 kg, give 12.5 to 25 mg per kg, divided into 4 doses a day. If you cannot weigh the person, dose by age:
Under 1 year: give 20 mg by mouth, 4 times a day.
1 to 5 years: give 30 mg by mouth, 4 times a day.
6 to 12 years: give 80 mg by mouth, 4 times a day.
Over 12 years: give 125 to 250 mg by mouth, 4 times a day.

For an infected wound, give the dose above for 5 to 7 days. If the wound is very dirty, also give metronidazole (page 99).

For a burn that is infected, give the dose above for 5 to 7 days. If it is a deep burn, or the person has a fever, give the dose above for 10 to 14 days.

Injectable penicillin, penicillin G

Injectable penicillin is used for certain severe infections, including infections from wounds.

Injectable penicillin comes in different forms. The main difference is how long the medicine lasts in the body and how quickly it works: short-acting, intermediate-acting, or long-acting.

How to use

BENZATHINE BENZYLPENICILLIN, BENZATHINE PENICILLIN G (long-acting)
Inject only in the muscle (IM), not in the vein (IV).

For a newborn baby with tetanus, inject 100,000 Units (U or IU) in the thigh muscle on the way to a hospital or health center.

PROCAINE PENICILLIN, PROCAINE BENZYLPENICILLIN (intermediate-acting)
Inject only in the muscle (IM), not in the vein (IV).

➡ Give 50,000 Units (U or IU) per kg per day. If you cannot weigh the person, dose by age:

2 months to 3 years: inject 150,000 Units, 1 time a day for 10 to 15 days.
4 to 7 years: inject 300,000 Units, 1 time a day for 10 to 15 days.
8 to 12 years: inject 600,000 Units, 1 time a day for 10 to 15 days.
Over 12 years: inject 600,000 to 2,400,000 Units, 1 time a day for 10 to 14 days.

Do not give to babies under 2 months unless no other penicillin or ampicillin is available. If this is your only choice, inject 50,000 Units, 1 time a day for 10 to 15 days.

Do not give children more than 1,200,000 Units in a day.

Other antibiotics

Erythromycin

Erythromycin works against many of the same infections as penicillin and can be used by those who are allergic to penicillins. For many infections, it can also be used in place of tetracycline. It can also be used for diphtheria and pertussis (whooping cough).

Side effects

Erythromycin often causes nausea and diarrhea, especially in children. Do not use for more than 2 weeks as it may cause jaundice.

How to use

➡ Give 30 to 50 mg per kg each day, divided into 2 to 4 doses a day. If you cannot weigh the person, dose by age:
Newborns up to 1 month old: give 62 mg, 3 times a day for 7 to 10 days.
1 month to 2 years: give 125 mg, 3 or 4 times a day for 7 to 10 days.
2 to 8 years: give 250 mg, 3 or 4 times a day for 7 to 10 days.
Over 8 years: give 250 to 500 mg, 4 times a day for 7 to 10 days.

Tetracycline and Doxycycline

Tetracycline and doxycycline are broad-spectrum antibiotics and fight many different kinds of bacteria. They work well when given by mouth (and are very painful when injected, so they should not be given that way). There are more infections that are now resistant to these medicines so they are not used as much as they once were, but they are still useful for fighting some infections.

Doxycycline and tetracycline can be used interchangeably. But doxycycline is usually a better choice because less is needed each day and it has fewer side effects.

Side effects

Heartburn, stomach cramps, diarrhea, and yeast infections are common.

Important ⚠

- Pregnant women should not take these medicines, as they can damage or stain the baby's teeth and bones. For the same reason, children under 8 years old should take them only when there is no other effective antibiotic, and for short periods only. You can usually use erythromycin instead.
- Some people may develop a skin rash or get easily sunburned after spending time in the sun while taking these medicines, so stay out of the sun or wear a large hat.

How to use

TETRACYCLINE

Avoid milk, iron pills, and antacids for 2 hours before or after taking tetracycline. They will make the medicine less effective.

Take tetracycline on an empty stomach, at least 1 hour before or 2 hours after meals.

For most infections

➡ Give 25 to 50 mg per kg each day, divided into 4 doses a day. If you cannot weigh the person, dose by age:

8 to 12 years: give 125 mg, 4 times a day for 7 to 10 days.
Over 12 years: give 250 to 500 mg, 4 times a day for 7 to 10 days.

DOXYCYCLINE

Doxycycline is taken twice a day (instead of 4 times a day like tetracycline).

Avoid milk, iron pills, and antacids for 2 hours before or after taking doxycycline. They will make the medicine less effective.

Take doxycycline on an empty stomach, at least 1 hour before or 2 hours after meals.

For most infections

➡ Give 2 mg per kg in each dose, but do not give more than 100 mg per dose or 200 mg a day. Give once or twice a day. Or dose by age:
8 to 12 years: give 50 mg twice a day, for 7 to 10 days.
Over 12 years: give 100 mg twice a day, for 7 to 10 days.

For animal bites, give the dose above for 3 to 5 days. Also give metronidazole (page 99) or clindamycin (page 98).

Cotrimoxazole, sulfamethoxazole with trimethoprim, TMP-SMX

Cotrimoxazole, a combination of 2 antibiotics, is inexpensive and fights a wide range of infections. It is an important medicine for people with HIV and can prevent the many infections that come as a result of HIV infection.

Important ⚠

Avoid giving cotrimoxazole to babies less than 6 weeks old and to women in the last 3 months of pregnancy. Allergy to this medicine is common. Signs of allergic reaction are fever, difficulty breathing, or rash. Stop giving cotrimoxazole if a rash develops or if you think there may be an allergy.

How to use

Cotrimoxazole comes in different strengths of each of the 2 medicines it contains. So it may say 200/40 (meaning 200 mg sulfamethoxazole and 40 mg trimethoprim) or 400/80 or 800/160. Sometimes a dose is described only in terms of the amount of trimethoprim (the second number).

For most infections

→ **6 weeks to 5 months:** give sulfamethoxazole 100 mg + trimethoprim 20 mg, 2 times a day for 5 days.
   6 months to 5 years: give sulfamethoxazole 200 mg + trimethoprim 40 mg, 2 times a day for 5 days.
   6 to 12 years: give sulfamethoxazole 400 mg + trimethoprim 80 mg, 2 times a day for 5 days.
   Over 12 years: give sulfamethoxazole 800 mg + trimethoprim 160 mg, 2 times a day for 5 days.

For animal bites, give the amount above for 3 to 5 days. Also give metronidazole (page 99) or clindamycin (page 98).

Clindamycin

Clindamycin is another antibiotic used to treat many kinds of bacterial infections. It is especially useful for treating infections that have become resistant to penicillin such as skin infections and abscesses.

Important ⚠

If you develop diarrhea that is watery or bloody while taking clindamycin, stop taking it immediately. This can be a sign of dangerous infection caused by the antibiotic. Because the drug can pass through breast milk and harm a baby, avoid giving to a breastfeeding woman.

How to use

Give clindamycin by mouth.

➡ **Under 3 years:** give 37.5 to 75 mg, 3 times a day.
3 to 7 years: give 75 to 150 mg, 3 times a day.
8 to 12 years: give 150 to 300 mg, 3 times a day.
Over 12 years: give 150 to 450 mg, 3 times a day.

For animal bites, give the dose above for 3 to 5 days. Also give another medicine such as doxycycline (page 96), cotrimoxazole (page 97) OR penicillin V (page 92).

For an infected wound, give the dose above for 5 to 7 days.

For a burn that is infected, give the dose above for 5 to 7 days. If it is a deep burn, or the person also has a fever, give the dose above for 10 to 14 days.

For a bone that has broken through the skin (open fracture), give the dose above for 5 to 7 days. If the wound is very dirty, also give ciprofloxacin (page 100).

For knife or gunshot wound, give the dose above for 10 to 14 days.

Metronidazole

Metronidazole is effective at fighting certain bacteria and infections, used by itself or in combination with other antibiotics.

Side effects

Nausea, cramps, and diarrhea are common. Taking with food may help. Sometimes it causes a metallic taste in the mouth or a headache.

Important ⚠

Do not give metronidazole in the first 3 months of pregnancy because it may cause birth defects. Also avoid giving metronidazole later in pregnancy and while breastfeeding unless it is the only effective medicine and is definitely needed. Do not drink alcohol while taking metronidazole or until 2 days after you finish taking it. Drinking alcohol while taking metronidazole causes severe nausea. Do not use metronidazole if you have liver problems.

How to use

→ Give 30 mg per kg, divided into 4 doses a day. If you cannot weigh the person, dose by age:
Under 1 year: give 37 mg, 4 times a day.
1 to 5 years: give 75 mg, 4 times a day.
6 to 12 years: give 150 mg, 4 times a day.
Over 12 years: Give 500 mg, 3 or 4 times a day. Do not give more than 4 g in
24 hours.

For an infected wound, give the dose above for 5 to 7 days. Also give dicloxacillin (page 93) OR cephalexin (page 102).

For a wound likely to be infected with tetanus, along with medicines to prevent tetanus (page 104), antibiotics are sometimes given. For example give the dose above for 7 to 10 days.

For animal bites, give the dose above for 3 to 5 days. Also give another medicine such as doxycycline (page 96), cotrimoxazole (page 97), OR penicillin V (page 92).

For a bone that has broken through the skin (open fracture), give the dose above for 5 to 7 days. Also give ceftriaxone (page 101), cephalexin (page 102) OR cloxacillin (page 92).

Ciprofloxacin

Ciprofloxacin is a broad spectrum antibiotic of the quinolone family. It works against a lot of different infections of the skin, bones, digestive tract, and urinary tract (bladder and kidneys). There are more infections becoming resistant to ciprofloxacin depending on where you live. Only use it against the infections for which it is specifically recommended in your area. It is not a good antibiotic for children.

Side effects

Nausea, diarrhea, vomiting, headache, dizziness, rash, or yeast infections.

Important ⚠

• Do not use if you are pregnant or breastfeeding. Do not take with dairy products such as milk or cheese.

• Rarely, ciprofloxacin damages the tendons. Except for a few specific situations, it should not be given to children under 16 because their tendons are still developing. If you have pain in your calves when taking this medicine, stop taking it immediately.

How to use

For most infections

➡ Give 250 to 750 mg, twice a day until 24 hours after signs of infection are gone.

For sepsis, give the dose above for 2 to 3 days after signs of infection are gone. Also give clindamycin (page 98).

For a bone that has broken through the skin (open fracture), give the dose above for 5 to 7 days. Also give clindamycin (page 98).

For a burn that is infected, give the dose above for 5 to 7 days. If it is a deep burn, or the person also has a fever, give the dose above for 10 to 14 days.

Ceftriaxone

Ceftriaxone is in the cephalosporin antibiotic family. Cephalosporins are antibiotics that work against many kinds of bacteria. They are often expensive and not widely available. However, they generally have fewer risks and side effects than many other antibiotics and can be useful in treating certain serious diseases.

Ceftriaxone is used against serious infections including sepsis and meningitis, and for infections resistant to penicillin. Only use ceftriaxone to treat the specific infections for which it is recommended in your area.

Ceftriaxone is especially useful for gonorrhea, including gonorrhea infection of the newborn's eyes but otherwise should not be given to newborns under 1 week old and should be avoided in babies under 1 month old.

Important ⚠

Do not give this medicine to someone who is allergic to other cephalosporin antibiotics.

Do not give to a baby less than 1 week old, except as treatment for gonorrhea in the eyes. Do not use if there is jaundice.

How to use

Ceftriaxone cannot be taken by mouth. When injecting, put the needle deep in the muscle. It can be painful to inject, so mix with 1% lidocaine (page 124) if you know how.

➡ Give 50 to 100 mg per kg each day, divided into 2 doses a day. If you cannot weigh the person, dose by age:
   1 to 3 months: inject 150 mg, twice a day.
   3 months to 1 year: inject 250 mg, twice a day.
   2 to 4 years: inject 400 mg, twice a day.
   5 to 12 years: inject 625 mg, twice a day.
   Over 12 years: inject 1 to 2 grams, once a day. Do not give more than 4 grams in 24 hours.

For a bone that has broken through the skin (open fracture), give the dose above for 5 to 7 days. If the wound is dirty, also give metronidazole (page 99).

For sepsis, give the dose above until 2 to 3 days after signs of infection are gone. If the wound is dirty, or there is no improvement 24 hours after starting ceftriaxone, also give metronidazole (page 99).

Cephalexin

Cephalexin is in the cephalosporin antibiotic family. Cephalosporins are powerful antibiotics that work against many kinds of bacteria. They are often expensive and not widely available. However, they generally have fewer risks and side effects than many other antibiotics and can be useful in treating certain serious diseases.

Side effects

Diarrhea that is watery or bloody, fever, sore throat, headache, red skin rash with blistering or peeling, dark colored urine, confusion or weakness.

Important ⚠

Do not give this medicine to someone who is allergic to other cephalosporin antibiotics.

How to use

→ Give 50 mg per kg each day, divided into 4 doses a day. Do not give more than 4000 mg in 24 hours. If you cannot weigh the person, dose by age:
Under 6 months: give 100 mg, 4 times a day.
6 months to 2 years: give 125 mg, 4 times a day.
3 to 5 years: give 250 mg, 4 times a day.
6 to 12 years: give 375 mg, 4 times a day.
Over 12 years: give 500 mg, 4 times a day.

For an infected wound, give the dose above for 5 to 7 days. If the wound is very dirty, also give metronidazole (page 99).

For a burn that is infected, give the dose above for 5 to 7 days. If it is a deep burn, or the person has a fever, give the dose above for 10 to 14 days.

For a bone that has broken through the skin (open fracture), give the dose above for 5 to 7 days. If the wound is very dirty, also give metronidazole (page 99).

For knife or gunshot wound, give the dose above for 10 to 14 days. If the wound is dirty or in the abdomen, also give metronidazole (page 99).

Gentamicin

Gentamicin is a very strong antibiotic of the aminoglycoside family. It can only be given by injection or IV (in the vein). This drug can damage the kidneys and the hearing, so it should only be used in emergencies.

Important ⚠

Gentamicin must be given in the exactly correct dose. Giving too much can cause kidney damage or permanent deafness. It is best to dose by weight. And do not give gentamicin for more than 10 days.

How to use

Inject into the muscle or the vein.

For sepsis

→ **6 months to 12 years:** inject 2.5 mg per kg, 3 times a day.
Over 12 years: inject 1 to 1.7 mg per kg, 3 times a day.

Medicines to Prevent Tetanus

Some wounds can cause tetanus (page 29) unless the person has already had the necessary vaccinations. Antitetanus immunoglobulin and the tetanus vaccine are 2 medicines given by injection that prevent tetanus after a wound. One or both are needed depending on the seriousness of the wound and whether the person is up-to-date with tetanus vaccinations. Give the necessary medicines as soon as possible. Do not wait for signs of tetanus.

A person is **up-to-date** with tetanus vaccines, when:
- they had all 6 doses (a series of 3 as a baby, and later at least 3 boosters).
  OR
- they had the series of 3 doses as a baby and at least one booster within the last 10 years.

To know which medicines are needed to prevent tetanus after a wound, you need to know if the person has been vaccinated against tetanus and when. Many people do not know if they have had these vaccines. If their vaccination history is unknown, give medicines as if they have not been vaccinated.

Type of wound	Tetanus vaccination history	
	Complete vaccination (3 or more doses)	**Incomplete vaccination (less than 3 doses) or vaccination status unknown**
Minor and clean	*last dose or most recent booster in the last 10 years:* no medicine needed	start or complete tetanus vaccine series (page 106)
	last dose or most recent booster more than 10 years ago: give 1 dose tetanus vaccine (page 106)	start or complete tetanus vaccine series (page 106)
Deep or dirty	*last dose or most recent booster in the last 5 years:* no medicine needed	start or complete tetanus vaccine series (page 106)
	last dose or most recent booster 5 to 10 years ago: give 1 dose tetanus vaccine (page 106)	start or complete tetanus vaccine series (page 106)
	last dose or most recent booster more than 10 years ago: give 1 dose tetanus vaccine (page 106)	start or complete tetanus vaccine series (page 106) AND give 1 dose antitetanus immunoglobulin (page 106)

If the person has HIV or another illness that lowers their immunity, give antitetanus immunoglobulin for any wound, even a minor one. If they are not up-to-date with their tetanus vaccination, give them the tetanus vaccine too.

Tetanus vaccine

- Vaccines to prevent tetanus often come combined with vaccines to prevent other illnesses. Abbreviations for such vaccines include DPT, Tdap, Td, and Dt.
- The DPT vaccine protects against diphtheria, pertussis, and tetanus and by 6 months old, babies need a series of 3 injections of this vaccine.
- Older children get 3 booster injections of DTP or another combination vaccine to prevent diphtheria and tetanus (such as Td or Dt).
- Receiving all 6 doses of these vaccines against tetanus (the series of 3 and then 3 boosters) gives protection from tetanus for decades.
- People who did not receive all 6 doses or did not have a dose within the last 10 years may need a booster vaccine.
- Giving the vaccine against tetanus to a pregnant woman whose vaccinations are not up-to-date helps protect both the woman and her newborn baby from tetanus.

Antitetanus immunoglobulin (human tetanus immune globulin, *HyperTET*)

If a person is not up-to-date with their tetanus vaccination (the series of 3 injections and at least 3 boosters, or 1 booster within the past 10 years), then give antitetanus immunoglobulin as soon as possible after a wound that could cause tetanus. If giving both the tetanus vaccine and the antitetanus immunoglobulin at the same time, give these in separate needles and do not inject antitetanus immunoglobulin in the same place on the body where you inject the tetanus vaccine. This will stop the vaccination from working.

Side effects

There may be pain and tenderness where the injection was given.

Important ⚠

Antitetanus immunoglobulin can cause a severe allergic reaction for some people. Always have epinephrine (adrenaline) available in case of an allergic reaction (page 112).

Some live virus vaccines, including those preventing measles, rubella, and tuberculosis, should not be given for 3 months after someone has received antitetanus immunoglobulin because it may make the other vaccines less effective.

How to use

Inject the medicine deep into the muscle.

For a wound less than 24 hours old
➡ Inject 250 Units one time only.

For a wound more than 24 hours old, or a wound that is very likely to be infected with tetanus
➡ Inject 500 Units one time only.

Also give an antibiotic such as metronidazole (page 99). For newborns with tetanus, give benzathine benzylpenicillin (page 94).

Medicines for Animal Bites

Clean animal bites well with soap and water. Give antibiotics because animal bites are especially likely to become infected.

➡ Amoxicillin with clavulanic acid (page 91) is the best choice for treating animal bites.

➡ If you do not have amoxicillin with clavulanic acid, use 2 antibiotics:

Give one of these: doxycycline (page 96), cotrimoxazole (page 97), or penicillin V (page 92)

AND, one of these: metronidazole (page 99) or clindamycin (page 98).

If the bite was from a dog, a bat, or another animal that could have rabies, also give rabies vaccine and rabies immunoglobulin if needed (see below).

Rabies vaccine and rabies immunoglobulin

Where there are animals with rabies, any animal bite or scratch breaking the skin will need thorough cleaning with soap and water for at least 15 minutes, a series of rabies vaccine injections, and, if the rabies risk is high, also an injection of rabies immunoglobulin (see "Animal bites," page 25). Even if there is no rabies immunoglobulin available, washing the skin thoroughly and giving the series of rabies vaccine can prevent rabies.

Using rabies vaccine

Inject the complete vial of vaccine (either 0.5 ml or 1 ml depending on the vaccine manufacturer) into the upper arm muscle on the day of the bite, and then again on days 3, and 7. Then, a fourth injection is given between day 14 (2 weeks) and 28 (4 weeks) after the bite. For a child 2 years or younger, give injections in the upper thigh.

Using rabies immunoglobulin

There are two forms of rabies immunoglobulin, one made from human serum (HRIG) and one made from horse serum (ERIG). HRIG is safer.

When giving rabies immunoglobulin, also give rabies vaccine, but use a different clean needle and inject in a different place on the body.

Important ⚠

Rabies immunoglobulin can cause a severe allergic reaction for some people. Always have epinephrine (adrenaline) available in case of an allergic reaction (page 112).

How to use 📝

Inject rabies immunoglobulin in and around the cleaned wound. If there are several wounds and the amount of rabies immunoglobulin you have is not enough to inject into each one, add buffered saline solution to double the amount of liquid. Then the person will still receive the correct dose and all wounds will receive some medicine.

If using Human Rabies Immune Globulin (HRIG)
→ Inject 20 Units per kg one time.

If using Equine Rabies Immune Globulin (ERIG)
→ Inject 40 Units per kg one time.

Medicines for Burns

Burns can be very painful. Give strong pain medicines such as codeine (page 122) OR morphine (page 123), especially before cleaning or changing the dressing on a burn.

Burns are very likely to get infected, so give an antibiotic such as dicloxacillin (page 93), clindamycin (page 98), cephalexin (page 102), OR ciprofloxacin (page 100) if there are any signs of infection.

As the burn heals, give an antihistamine like chlorpheniramine (below) OR diphenhydramine (page 111) to calm the itching.

Give a tetanus vaccine if the person's tetanus vaccination is not up-to-date (pages 104 to 107).

If the person was in a fire and inhaled a lot of smoke, salbutamol can help them to breathe more easily (page 113).

Medicines for Allergy or Itching: Antihistamines

Itching, sneezing, and rashes caused by allergy can usually be treated with antihistamines. Any antihistamine works about as well as any other. So if you do not have chlorpheniramine or diphenhydramine, use another antihistamine in the right dose (this will vary for each drug). All antihistamines make people drowsy, but some more than others.

These drugs are not helpful for the common cold.

Antihistamines should be avoided during pregnancy. If they must be given, choose a "first generation" antihistamine such as chlorpheniramine or diphenhydramine, and give with plenty of water.

For a severe allergic reaction where there is difficulty breathing, epinephrine (adrenaline) is needed as well as antihistamines (page 111).

Chlorpheniramine, chlorphenamine

Chlorpheniramine is an antihistamine that reduces itching, sneezing, rashes, and other problems caused by allergies. It can be used after an insect bite, a mild allergy to a food or a medicine, or for "hay fever" (sneezing and itchy eyes from pollen in the air).

Side effects

Sleepiness (but this is less likely than with other antihistamines).

Important ⚠

Do not give to pregnant women unless necessary. Do not give during an asthma attack.

How to use

→ **1 to 2 years:** give 1 mg, 2 times a day until the child feels better.
3 to 5 years: give 1 mg, every 4 to 6 hours until the child feels better.
6 to 12 years: give 2 mg, every 4 to 6 hours until the child feels better.
Over 12 years: give 4 mg, every 4 to 6 hours until the person feels better.

For severe allergic reaction

First inject epinephrine (page 112). Follow with chlorpheniramine by mouth in the doses listed above to help prevent the reaction from coming back when the epinephrine wears off.

Diphenhydramine

Diphenhydramine is an antihistamine that reduces itching, sneezing, rashes, and other problems caused by allergies. It can be used after an insect bite, a mild food or drug allergy, or for "hay fever" (sneezing and itchy eyes from pollen in the air).

Side effects

Sleepiness.

Important

- Diphenhydramine may cause dizziness, sleepiness, or blurred vision. Do not drive or operate machinery if using this medicine. Drinking alcohol may increase the sleepiness caused by diphenhydramine.

- Do not give to newborn babies or women who are breastfeeding. It is best not to give diphenhydramine to pregnant women unless necessary.

- Do not give during an asthma attack.

How to use

The dose is the same for giving diphenhydramine by mouth or as an injection into the muscle.

➡ **2 to 5 years:** give 6 mg every 4 to 6 hours. Do not give more than 37 mg per day.
6 to 11 years: give 12 to 25 mg every 4 to 6 hours. Do not give more than 150 mg per day.
Over 12 years: give 25 to 50 mg every 4 to 6 hours. Do not give more than 400 mg per day.

For severe allergic reaction

First inject epinephrine (page 112). Following with diphenhydramine in the doses below will help prevent the reaction from coming back when the epinephrine wears off.

➡ **2 to 11 years:** give 1 to 2 mg per kg, every 6 hours. If you cannot weigh the child, use the doses by age listed above, and give the larger amount. Do not give more than 50 mg at one time, or 300 mg per day.
Over 12 years: give 25 to 50 mg, every 2 to 4 hours. Do not give more than 100 mg in 4 hours or 400 mg per day.

Epinephrine (adrenaline)

Epinephrine is used for severe allergic reaction (anaphylaxis) to medicines, foods, insect stings or bites, or other things that cause a severe allergic reaction. It helps reverse the effects such as difficulty breathing, wheezing, severe skin itching, and hives.

Side effects

Fear, restlessness, nervousness, tension, headaches, dizziness, increased heart rate.

Important ⚠

Epinephrine often comes in ampules of 1 mg per 1 ml liquid. Epinephrine is also available in preloaded autoinjectors, but these come in different amounts. Be sure to read to see how much epinephrine is in your autoinjector to make sure you are giving the correct amount.

How to use

For severe allergic reaction
➡ Inject into the muscle in the outer part of the mid-thigh.

1 to 5 years: inject ¼ mg (0.25 mg).
6 to 12 years: inject ⅓ mg (0.33 mg).
Over 12 years: inject ½ mg (0.5 mg).

If needed, you can give a second dose in 5 to 15 minutes, and a third dose in 5 to 15 minutes after that. Do not give more than 3 doses.

After giving epinephrine, give an antihistamine such as chlorpheniramine (page 110) or diphenhydramine (page 111). This will help prevent the reaction from coming back when the epinephrine wears off.

Salbutamol (albuterol)

Salbutamol relaxes the muscles in the airway to increase air flow to the lungs. It is used to treat wheezing or shortness of breath from asthma or inhaling a lot of smoke from a fire.

Side effects

Trembling, nervousness, dizziness, fast heartbeat, and headaches.

How to use

➡ Give 2 puffs from an inhaler (200 micrograms) every 4 to 6 hours as needed. Use with a spacer for better effects.

It is OK to give more than the amounts listed above if the person feels they need it.

Medicines for Heart Attack

If you suspect someone is having a heart attack, give 1 tablet of aspirin right away (300 to 325 mg). Ask the person to chew it and swallow it with water. Even if you are not sure the person is having a heart attack, aspirin will do no harm. On the way to a hospital, give nitroglycerin if you have it. You can also give morphine to help with the pain and fear (page 123).

Nitroglycerin (Glyceryl trinitrate)

Nitroglycerin is used to treat chest pain from a heart attack. It helps to widen the blood vessels making it easier for the heart to pump blood.

Important ⚠

Do not give nitroglycerin to someone with low blood pressure or who has taken sildenafil (*Viagra*) in the last 24 hours. This combination of medicines can cause blood pressure to drop dangerously low, and can be deadly.

Side effects

May cause severe headache, feeling hot, or dizziness.

How to use

The person should sit or lie down, not stand up, in case they get dizzy.

➡ Give ½ mg (0.5 mg) tablet dissolved under the tongue, no more than 3 times, waiting 5 minutes between each tablet. If the chest pain and other signs go away, another tablet is not needed. Do not chew or swallow nitroglycerin tablets. As the tablet dissolves under the tongue, it tingles or even burns a little.

Medicines for Poisoning

Activated charcoal

Activated charcoal is a powder used to treat some poisonings such as certain pesticides and herbicides that have been swallowed. Activated charcoal prevents the poison from being absorbed by the body, so give it as soon as possible after being poisoned. Activated charcoal will not harm a person who was not poisoned, so give it even if you are not sure.

If you do not have activated charcoal, you can use powdered charcoal from burnt wood or even burnt bread or tortilla. Mix 1 tablespoon of powdered charcoal with warm water in a large glass. This is not as good as activated charcoal, but it still works.

Never use charcoal briquettes—they are poison!

Activated charcoal is **not** helpful for poisoning from:

- **corrosives** (such as ammonia, batteries, acids, drain cleaner, caustic soda, lye)
- **hydrocarbons** (such as gasoline, kerosene, turpentine, paint thinner, phenol, carbolic acid, camphor, pine oil)
- **cyanide** (used in mining, factory work, animal hide hair removal, rat poison)
- **ethanol**
- **iron** (iron tablets, multivitamins, or prenatal vitamins)
- **lithium** (found in medication to treat bipolar mental illness)
- **methanol** (found in varnish, paint thinner, fuel additives for cars)
- **mineral acids**
- **organic solvents** (found in paint thinner, glue solvents, nail polish remover, spot removers)

Side effects

Can cause black stools, vomiting, constipation, or diarrhea.

How to use

➡ Give as soon as possible after poisoning (or possible poisoning) with a full glass of water. The dose can be given again in 4 hours.
Under 1 year: give 10 to 25 g.
1 year to 12 years: give 25 to 50 g.
Over 12 years: give 50 g.

Atropine

Atropine is used to treat poisoning from certain pesticides, insecticides, or nerve gases. Only use atropine if the label on the pesticide container says to use atropine, or if it says the pesticide is a "cholinesterase inhibitor." The amount of atropine needed depends on how severe the poisoning is. Usually, a poisoning from a carbamate requires less medicine than if the poisoning is from an organophosphate.

Side effects

Sleepiness, feeling lightheaded, headaches, changes in thinking, and hard stools.

Important ⚠

Keep the person cool after giving atropine.

How to use

➡ Inject into the muscle.
Children: inject 0.02 to 0.05 mg per kg, every 5 to 10 minutes.
Adults: inject 2 mg, every 5 to 10 minutes.

Repeat dose every 5 to 10 minutes until the person can breathe more easily and their pupils have gotten bigger.

Deferoxamine

Deferoxamine helps treat iron poisoning by removing iron from the blood.

Side effects

Blurred vision and changes in thinking.

Important ⚠

Do not give to someone with kidney disease or if the person cannot urinate. Do not give to children under 3 years old.

How to use

➡ Inject slowly into the muscle. Inject 50 mg per kg every 6 hours. Do not give more than 6 g in a day. If you cannot weigh the person, dose by age:
   3 to 5 years: slowly inject 500 mg, every 6 hours, for 1 day (4 times).
   5 to 12 years: slowly inject 1000 mg, every 6 hours, for 1 day (4 times).
   Over 12 years: slowly inject every 6 hours for 1 day (4 times) as follows: The first 2 times give 2000 mg, then use half the dose, 1000 mg, for the next 2 times.

Acetylcysteine

Give acetylcysteine as soon as possible after taking too much paracetamol or acetaminophen. Too much paracetamol or acetaminophen is over 7,000 mg for an adult, and over 140 mg per kg for a child.

   Acetylcysteine has a strong smell. Mixing it with juice helps the person tolerate it.

How to use

For paracetamol (acetaminophen) overdose

➡ Give the first dose of acetylcysteine at 140 mg per kg by mouth. Wait 4 hours then give half this amount for the second dose (70 mg per kg by mouth). Continue giving the dose of 70 mg per kg every 4 hours, 16 more times. This makes a total of 18 doses during a 3-day period (72 hours). If the person vomits within 1 hour of taking the medicine, give the dose again.

Naloxone

Naloxone is used to treat an overdose from opioids such as morphine, heroin, fentanyl, methadone, opium, oxycodone, codeine, and other strong pain medicines. Give naloxone until the person is breathing well on their own. The treatment can wear off, so you may need to give another dose in 20 minutes if the person starts to have difficulty breathing again.

Side effects

Nausea, vomiting, and sweating. Extreme discomfort.

How to use

→ **Under 5 years or child weighs less than 20 kg:** inject 0.1 mg per kg into the muscle every 2 to 3 minutes as needed, but do not give more than 2 mg in total.
Over 5 years or weighs more than 20 kg: inject ½ to 2 mg in the muscle. If needed, repeat the dose every 2 to 3 minutes, but do not give more than 10 mg in total.

Sodium nitrite

Sodium nitrite is used to treat cyanide poisoning together with sodium thiosulfate. It must be injected into the vein. Only do this if you know how.

How to use

→ Slowly inject sodium nitrite into the vein over 5 to 20 minutes.
Under 12 years: inject 4 to 10 mg per kg into the vein. Do not give more than 300 mg.
Over 12 years: inject 300 mg into the vein.

Follow with an injection of sodium thiosulfate. See page 119 for doses.

Sodium thiosulfate

Sodium thiosulfate is used to treat cyanide poisoning along with an injection of sodium nitrite. It must be injected into the vein. Only do this if you know how.

How to use

➡ Slowly inject sodium thiosulfate into the vein over 10 minutes.
  Under 12 years: inject 400 mg per kg into the vein.
  Over 12 years: inject 12.5 g into the vein.

Medicines for Pain

Medicines for mild pain and lowering fever include paracetamol (the safest and best medicine to use for children), aspirin, and ibuprofen. Aspirin and ibuprofen also reduce inflammation (swelling). Reducing swelling will calm pain and help heal injuries such as a twisted or sprained ankle. For children with fevers and viral infections, give paracetamol and avoid aspirin.

Do not give more than the recommended dose of these medicines. Too much aspirin or ibuprofen can cause stomach ulcers. Too much paracetamol can be poisonous. For high fever or very strong pain, avoid using too much of any one pain medicine by using both paracetamol and ibuprofen in the correct doses and intervals.

Paracetamol, acetaminophen

Paracetamol is a good, affordable medicine for fever and mild pain.

Important ⚠

Do not take more than the recommended amount. Too much is poisonous to the liver and can kill. Keep this medicine out of the reach of children, especially if you have it as a sweetened syrup.

Cold medicines often contain paracetamol, so do not give them if you are also giving paracetamol or you may give too much.

How to use

→ Give 10 to 15 mg per kg, every 4 to 6 hours. Do not give more than 5 times in 24 hours. If you cannot weigh the person, dose by age:
Under 1 year: give 62 mg (half of ¼ of a 500 mg tablet), every 4 to 6 hours.
1 to 2 years: give 125 mg (¼ of a 500 mg tablet), every 4 to 6 hours.
3 to 7 years: give 250 mg (½ of a 500 mg tablet), every 4 to 6 hours.
8 to 12 years: give 375 mg (¾ of a 500 mg tablet), every 4 to 6 hours.
Over 12 years: give 500 mg to 1000 mg, every 4 to 6 hours, but do not give more than 4000 mg in a day.

Ibuprofen

Ibuprofen relieves muscle pain, joint pain, and headache, and lowers fever.

Side effects

Ibuprofen can cause a stomachache, but taking it with milk or food lessens that problem.

Important ⚠

Do not take ibuprofen if you are allergic to aspirin. Some people who are allergic to one are also allergic to the other. Do not give ibuprofen for stomach pain or indigestion. Ibuprofen is acidic and may make the problem worse. For the same reason, people with stomach ulcers should never use ibuprofen. Do not give ibuprofen to babies younger than 6 months, and do not give to pregnant women in their last 3 months of pregnancy.

How to use

3 to 11 months: 50 mg, 3 times a day
1 to 3 years: 100 mg, 3 times a day
4 to 6 years: 150 mg, 3 times a day
7 to 9 years: 200 mg, 3 times a day

10 to 11 years: 300 mg, 3 times a day
12 years and older: 300 to 400 mg, 3 times a day

For children under 12 years, do not give more than 30 mg per kg in 1 day. For people 12 years and older, do not give more than 1200 mg total in 1 day.

Aspirin (acetylsalicylic acid)

Aspirin is a good, affordable medicine for fever and mild pain.

Side effects

Aspirin can cause stomach pain or heartburn. To avoid this, take aspirin with milk, a little bicarbonate of soda, or a lot of water—or together with meals.

Important ⚠

- Do not give aspirin for stomach pain or indigestion. Aspirin is acidic and may make the problem worse. For the same reason, people with stomach ulcers should never use aspirin.
- Do not give more than 1 dose of aspirin to a dehydrated person until he begins to urinate well.
- Do not give aspirin to people with asthma, children younger than 1 year old, or children with flu signs. If possible, avoid giving to children younger than 12 years old and use ibuprofen or paracetamol instead.
- Keep aspirin where children cannot reach it. Large amounts can poison them.
- Do not give to pregnant women.

How to use

Over 12 years: give 300 to 600 mg, every 4 to 6 hours.
Do not give more than 4000 mg a day.

For heart attack

➡ Give 300 to 325 mg by mouth immediately.
Chew it up and swallow it.

Codeine (codeine sulfate)

Codeine is a medicine for pain in the opiate family. It is used to treat severe pain. Only use codeine when milder pain medicines do not work.

Side effects

May cause constipation (difficulty passing stools) and temporary inability to pass urine. May also cause nausea, vomiting, itching, and headaches.

Important ⚠

- Codeine is a habit-forming (addictive) drug. Avoid long-term or frequent use.
- Do not drink alcohol while using codeine as it can cause dangerous side effects and even death.
- Codeine can affect your thinking and reactions while taking it. Be careful when driving or doing other things that require you to be alert.
- Reduce the dose over time to stop taking it. Stopping all at once can cause uncomfortable withdrawal symptoms.
- Do not use codeine if you have ever had an allergic reaction to morphine.
- Do not use codeine if you are pregnant or breastfeeding.

How to use

➡ Give codeine along with food.
3 to 6 years: give ½ to 1 mg per kg by mouth, every 4 to 6 hours.
7 to 12 years: give 15 to 30 mg by mouth, every 4 to 6 hours.
Over 12 years: give 15 to 60 mg by mouth, every 4 to 6 hours. Do not give more than 360 mg per day.

Morphine (morphine sulfate, morphine hydrochloride)

Morphine is medicine for pain in the opiate family used to treat moderate to severe pain.

Important ⚠

- Morphine is a habit-forming (addictive) drug. Avoid long-term or frequent use.
- Do not drink alcohol while using morphine as it can cause dangerous side effects and even death.
- Morphine can affect your thinking and reactions while taking it. Be careful when driving or doing other things that require you to be alert.
- Reduce the dose over time to stop taking it. Stopping all at once can cause uncomfortable withdrawal symptoms.
- Do not use morphine if you have ever had an allergic reaction to codeine.
- Do not use morphine if you are pregnant or breastfeeding.

How to use

For moderate to severe pain

→ **Under 6 months:** give 0.1 mg per kg by mouth, every 3 to 4 hours. If you cannot weigh the baby, give 0.5 mg by mouth, every 3 to 4 hours.
Over 6 months: give 0.2 to 0.5 mg per kg by mouth, every 4 to 6 hours as needed. If you cannot weigh the person, dose by age:
6 months to 1 year: give 2 mg by mouth, every 4 to 6 hours.
1 to 5 years: give 3 mg by mouth, every 4 to 6 hours.
6 to 12 years: give 8 mg by mouth, every 4 to 6 hours.
Over 12 years: give 10 to 30 mg by mouth, every 4 hours as needed.

For heart attack

→ Slowly inject 10 mg into the muscle over 5 minutes (2 mg per minute). Inject another 5 to 10 mg if necessary.

Medicines for Numbing

Lidocaine, Lignocaine

Lidocaine is an anesthetic that can be injected around the edges of a wound to make the area numb so it will not hurt. This is useful before cleaning or stitching up a wound.

Lidocaine often comes in a 2% solution which is 20 mg of lidocaine per ml. If you have a different percent (%) solution, adjust the amount you use.

How to use

➡ Slowly inject into and under the skin around where you are going to cut or sew, at points about 1 cm apart. Inject the lidocaine close to the surface of the skin. Use about 1 ml of lidocaine for each 2 cm of skin. Do not use more than 20 ml.

Anti-anxiety Medicines

Diazepam

Diazepam can be used to relax muscles and calm the person. It can also be used to stop a single seizure. For people with ongoing seizures (epilepsy), use a different medicine, one that can be taken every day.

Side effects

Sleepiness.

Important ⚠️

* Too much diazepam can slow down or stop breathing. **Do not give more than the recommended dose and do not give more than 2 doses.**
* Diazepam is a habit-forming (addictive) drug. Avoid long-term or frequent use.
* Do not give during pregnancy or breastfeeding unless the woman has a seizure (for example, due to eclampsia).
* Do not inject diazepam unless you have experience or training to do so. It is very difficult to give safely by injection. Instead, during a seizure, you can put it into the rectum (see below).

How to use 🖐️

To relax muscles and calm a person

Give diazepam tablets by mouth 45 minutes before a painful procedure like pushing in a hernia or setting a bone.

➡ For children, give 0.2 to 0.3 mg per kg. If you cannot weigh the person, dose by age:
2 to 6 years: give 1 mg.
7 to 12 years: give 5 mg.
Over 12 years: give 10 mg.

For a seizure

➡ Use the liquid, the gel, or grind up 1 tablet and mix with water. Take the needle off a syringe, then draw up the medication. Lay the person on her side and use the needle-less syringe to put the medicine deep into her rectum. Then hold her buttocks together for 10 minutes to keep the medicine in.
Under 5 years: give 0.5 mg per kg, 1 time.
5 years and over: give 10 mg, 1 time.

If the seizure does not stop within 10 minutes after the first dose, give a second dose. Do not give more after that.

Lorazepam

Lorazepam is very similar to diazepam. It can be used to relax muscles and calm the person. It can also be used to stop a single seizure. For people with ongoing seizures (epilepsy), use a different medicine, one that can be taken every day.

Side effects

Sleepiness.

Important

- Too much lorazepam can slow down or stop breathing.
- Lorazepam is a habit-forming (addictive) drug. Avoid long-term or frequent use.
- Do not give during pregnancy or breastfeeding unless the woman has a seizure (for example, due to eclampsia).
- Do not inject lorazepam into a muscle or vein unless you have experience or training to do so. It is very difficult to give safely by injection. Instead, during a seizure, you can put it into the rectum (see "Diazepam, For a seizure," page 125).

How to use

To relax muscles and calm a person

➡ Give lorazepam tablets by mouth 45 minutes before a painful procedure like setting a bone.
1 month to 12 years: give 0.05 mg per kg, one time.
Over 12 years: give 1 to 2 mg, one time.

Other Books from Hesperian

Hesperian resources are available in English, Spanish, and a variety of other languages. See the Language Hub on our website (hesperian.org) to find materials in your language.

General Health Books

Where There Is No Doctor, perhaps the most widely used health care manual in the world, provides vital, easily understood information on how to diagnose, treat, and prevent common diseases. An emphasis is placed on prevention, including cleanliness, diet, vaccinations, and the important role of the individual and community in health care. 446 pages, paperback.

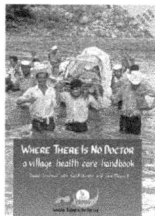

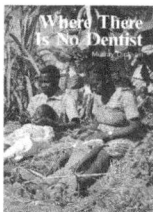

Where There Is No Dentist shows how to care for teeth and gums at home and in community and school settings, including prevention of dental issues through hygiene, nutrition, and education. The book also includes detailed and illustrated information on using dental equipment, placing fillings, taking out teeth, and material on HIV/AIDS and oral health. 248 pages, paperback.

Promoting Community Mental Health is a new concise guide offering innovative strategies and practical tools that people from all walks of life can use in their efforts to improve the emotional and physical health of their communities. Developed with input from 26 community-led groups across the US, this resource helps community organizers, health workers, faith groups, and individuals integrate mental health promotion into their work and lives. 200 pages, paperback.

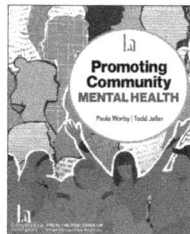

Reproductive and Women's Health

A Health Handbook for Women with Disabilities provides individuals and caregivers suggestions on caring for daily needs, healthy and safe sexual relationships, family planning, pregnancy and childbirth, and defense against violence, abuse, and stigma. This groundbreaking guide helps women with disabilities overcome barriers to poor health and advocate for better care. 384 pages, paperback.

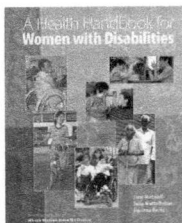

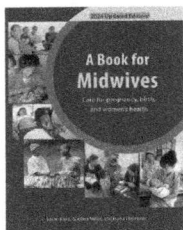

A Book for Midwives covers the essentials of care before, during, and after birth. A vital resource for practitioners, training programs, and anyone interested in safer birthing. Clearly written and illustrated, this book discusses preventing, managing, and treating obstetric complications, covers HIV in pregnancy, birth, and breastfeeding, and has expanded information on reproductive health care. 527 pages, paperback.

Where Women Have No Doctor combines self-help medical information with an understanding of the ways poverty, discrimination, and cultural beliefs limit women's health and access to care. Clearly written and with over 1000 drawings, this essential resource addresses health issues across the lifespan and considers issues specific to girls, older women, women with disabilities, and refugees. 583 pages, paperback.

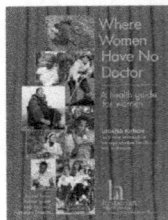

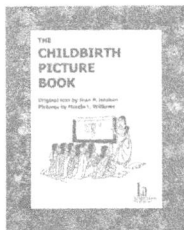

The Childbirth Picture Book provides a simple and complete guide to the basics of conception, pregnancy, childbirth, and breastfeeding. This short resource contains detailed line drawings depicting every step of the reproductive process.
68 pages, staple-bound booklet.

Health Organizing and Training

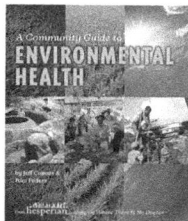

A Community Guide to Environmental Health
provides tools, knowledge, and inspiration to help
health promoters, activists, and community leaders
take charge of their environmental health. This
comprehensive guide supports urban and rural
communities and covers topics from toilets to toxics,
watershed management to waste management, and
agriculture to air pollution. Informative case studies,
impactful activities, and how-to instructions empower people to address
environmental health hazards where they live and work. 617 pages,
paperback.

Recruiting the Heart, Training the Brain tells the story of
how Latino Health Access developed its groundbreaking
promoter model of peer-to-peer outreach and education
in Santa Ana, California. Facing problems such as obesity
and diabetes, exacerbated by poverty and discrimination,
their strategies, advice, and accomplishments inspire
hope and change across an increasingly unhealthy
country. 280 pages, paperback.

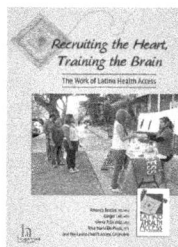

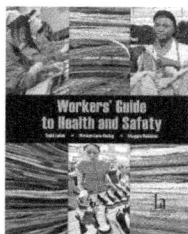

Workers' Guide to Health and Safety makes
occupational safety and health accessible to those most
affected by physical, social, and economic hazards—
the workers themselves. Actionable tools and strategies
support workers, supervisors, safety committees,
and labor relations courses to improve workplace
experiences and overall well-being for workers. The
insights and techniques are useful in any factory,
and especially in the garment, shoe, and electronics
industries.

See our website: hesperian.org
for many more books, booklets, and online resources.

Ordering from Hesperian

We provide bulk ordering discounts to bookstores, schools, non-profits, universities, and other organizations.

To purchase books, visit: store.hesperian.org
email: bookorders@hesperian.org
or call: 510-845-4507.

For more information about review or exam copies, or to apply for our Gratis Books Program which distributes free copies of Hesperian's community health books to health workers, teachers, and local leaders in low-income communities, please email: hesperian@hesperian.org or visit: hesperian.org.

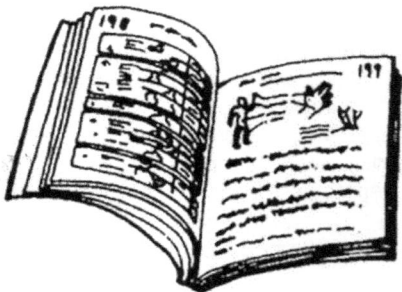

How are you using Hesperian resources?

Please tell us! We would love to hear how our resources enable you to make positive change.

hesperian.org/share-your-story

Notes

www.ingramcontent.com/pod-product-compliance
Lightning Source LLC
Chambersburg PA
CBHW030020290326
41934CB00005B/419